BESTMEDICINE

Alzheimer's Disease

Dr George Kassianos

Professor Susan Benbow

Dr Ian Greaves

Dr Steve Illiffe

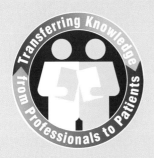

Foreword by Claire Rayner
President of the Patients Association

Managing Editor: Dr Scott Chambers
Medical Writers: Dr Eleanor Bull, Dr Rebecca Fox-Spencer, Dr Richard Clark
Editorial Controller: Emma Catherall
Operations Manager: Julia Potterton
Designer: Chris Matthews
Typesetter: Julie Smith
Indexer: Laurence Errington
Director – Online Business: Peter Llewellyn
Publishing Director: Julian Grover
Publisher: Stephen I'Anson

1 Bankside
Lodge Road
Long Hanborough
Oxfordshire
OX29 8LJ, UK
Tel: +44 (0)1993 885370
Fax: +44 (0)1993 881868
Email: *enquiries@bestmedicine.com*

www.bestmedicine.com
www.csfmedical.com

The content of *BESTMEDICINE* is the work of a number of authors and has been produced in line with our standard editorial procedures, including the peer review of the disease overview and the drug reviews, and the passing of the final manuscript for publication by the Managing Editor and the Editor-in-Chief or the Medical Editor. Whilst every effort has been made to ensure the accuracy of the information at the date of approval for publication, the Authors, the Publisher, the Editors and the Editorial Board accept no responsibility whatsoever for any errors or omissions or for any consequences arising from anything included in or excluded from *BESTMEDICINE*.

All reasonable effort is made to avoid infringement of copyright law, including the redrawing of figures adapted from other sources. Where copyright permission has been deemed necessary, attempts are made to gain appropriate permission from the copyright holder. However, the Authors, the Publisher, the Editors and the Editorial Board accept no personal responsibility for any infringement of copyright law howsoever made. Any queries regarding copyright approvals or permissions should be addressed to the Managing Editor.

You are strongly urged to consult your doctor before taking, stopping or changing any of the products reviewed or referred to in *BESTMEDICINE* or any other medication that has been prescribed or recommended by your doctor.

A catalogue record for this book is available from the British Library.

ISBN: 1-905064-93-4

Typeset by Creative, Langbank, Scotland.
Printed and bound in Wales.
Distributed by NBN International, Plymouth, Devon.

Contents

Foreword

Claire Rayner
President of The Patients Association

Patients and their families are rightly entitled to have access to good-quality, independent and reliable information concerning a diverse range of conditions and a wide variety of medications that are available to treat them. Indeed, there is a growing recognition amongst the majority of healthcare professionals that well-informed patients are more likely to adopt a more active role in the management of their illness and will therefore feel more satisfied with the care that they receive. Such an effect has the potential not only to directly benefit the patient and their families, but can also maximise limited healthcare resources within an already over-stretched NHS. However, at present access to this kind of information is limited, despite the fact that as many as one-in-four adults (12 million people in the UK alone) want ready access to this knowledge prior to visiting their doctor.

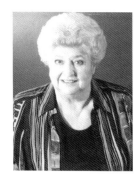

Photograph courtesy of
Amanda Rayner

    The importance of patient self-management is a key component of current NHS strategy. Indeed, this has been widely acknowledged in an NHS-led campaign called the Expert Patient Programme (*www.expertpatient.nhs.uk*). This is a self-management course which aims to give people the confidence, skills and knowledge to manage their condition better and take more control of their lives. The Expert Patient Programme defines an Expert Patient as one who has had the condition for long enough to have learnt the language doctors use.

    BESTMEDICINE aims to meet the information and educational needs of both patients and healthcare professionals alike. The information found in the *BESTMEDICINE* series will assist patients and their families to obtain the level of information they now need to understand and manage their medical condition in partnership with their doctor. However, as *BESTMEDICINE* draws much of its content from medical publications written by doctors for doctors, some readers may find these books rather challenging when they first approach them. Despite this, I strongly believe that the effort that you invest in reading this book will be fully repaid by the increased knowledge they you will gain about this condition. Indeed, the extensive glossary of terms that can be found within each book certainly makes understanding the text a great deal easier, and the Patient Notes section is also very informative and reassuringly written by a doctor for the less scientifically minded reader. *BESTMEDICINE* represents the world's first source of independent, unabridged medical information that will appeal to patients and their families as well as healthcare professionals. This development should be welcomed and applauded, and I would commend these books to you.

Claire Rayner, November 2004

Claire Rayner has been involved with the Patients Association for many years and has considerable expertise and experience from a professional background in nursing and journalism and her personal experience as a patient and carer. She is well known as a leading 'Agony Aunt' and as a medical correspondent for many popular magazines. Claire has also published articles in a number of professional journals, as well as over forty medical, nursing and patient advice books.

An introduction to *BESTMEDICINE*

The source: information for healthcare professionals

Over the years, it has become increasingly apparent that there is a dearth of drug-related information that is independently compiled and robustly reviewed, and which also acknowledges the challenges faced by healthcare professionals when applying evidence-based medicine whilst practising at the 'front line' of patient care. As such, many healthcare professionals feel a certain ambivalence towards the numerous drug review publications that are currently on offer and, indeed, many do not have confidence in the information that can be found within their pages. In response to the need for a more impartial information resource – one that is independent of the pharmaceutical industry and the health service – we developed a novel publication, which was launched to meet this perceived lack of independent information. This peer-reviewed publication is called *Drugs in Context* and was launched in May 2003 and is the source of much of what you will find in this edition of *BESTMEDICINE*.

Uniquely independent

Drugs in Context is unique in that it reviews the significant clinical and pharmacological evidence underpinning the use of a single drug, in the disease area(s) where it is used and the practice setting where it is most commonly prescribed. Over 50 issues are published each year covering numerous diseases and conditions. The principal goal of *Drugs in Context* is to become the definitive drug and disease management resource for all healthcare professionals. As such, over the coming years, the publication plans to review all of the significant drugs that are currently used in clinical practice.

Reliable and impartial information for patients too

In addition to the lack of impartial information for the healthcare professional, we also firmly believe that there is a significant and growing number of patients who are not served well in this regard either. Indeed, it is becoming apparent to us that many patients would welcome access to the same sources of information on drugs and diseases that their doctors and other healthcare professionals have access to.

There are numerous sources of information currently available to patients – ranging from leaflets and books to websites and other electronic media. However, despite their best intentions, the rigour and accuracy of many of these resources cannot be relied upon due to significant variation in the quality of the material. Perhaps the major problem facing a patient or a loved one who is hunting for specific information relating to a disease or the drug that has been prescribed by their doctor is that there is simply too much material available, making sifting through it to find a relevant fact akin to looking for a needle in a haystack! More importantly, many of these resources can often (albeit unintentionally) patronise the reader who has made every effort to actively seek out information that can serve to reassure themselves about the concerned illness and about the medication(s) prescribed for it.

Can knowledge be the '*BESTMEDICINE*'?

We firmly believe that by providing high quality education and information, patients and their families or carers are more likely to take an active role in the management of the disease or condition and, therefore, will be more likely gain further benefit from any course of treatment that is prescribed. This approach will provide benefits to everyone – the patient, their family and friends, the healthcare professionals involved in their care, and the NHS and the country as a whole! Indeed, such is the importance of patient education, that the NHS has launched an initiative emphasising the need for patients and carers of patients to assume a more active role in the management of chronic diseases via the acquisition of knowledge and skills related specifically to the particularly disease that is affecting them. This initiative is called the Expert Patients Programme (*www.expertpatients.nhs.uk*).

Filling the need for quality information

Many of our observations about the lack of quality education have underpinned the principles behind the launch of *BESTMEDICINE*, much of the content of which is drawn directly from the pages of *Drugs in Context*, as written by and for healthcare professionals. *BESTMEDICINE* aims to appeal primarily to the patient, loved-one or carer who wants to improve their knowledge of the disease in question, the evidence for and against the drugs available to treat the disease and the practical challenges faced by healthcare professionals in managing it.

A whole new language!

We fully acknowledge that a lot of medical terminology used in order to expedite communication amongst the medical community will be new to many of you, some terms may be difficult to pronounce and sometimes surplus to requirements. However, rather than significantly abridge the content and risk excluding something of importance to the reader, we have instead provided you with a comprehensive glossary of terms and what we hope will be helpful additional GP discussion pieces at the end of each section to aid understanding further. We have also provided you with an introduction to the processes underlying drug development and the key concepts in disease management which we hope you will also find informative and which we strongly recommend that you read before tackling the rest of this edition of *BESTMEDICINE*.

No secrets

By providing the same information to patients and their families as healthcare professionals we believe that *BESTMEDICINE* will help to foster better relationships between patients, their families and doctors and other healthcare professionals and ultimately may even improve treatment outcomes.

This edition is one of a number of unique collections of disease summaries and drug reviews that we will be making widely available over the coming months. You will find details about each issue as it is published at *www.bestmedicine.com*.

We do hope that you find this edition of *BESTMEDICINE* illuminating.

Dr George Kassianos, GP, Bracknell; Editor-in-Chief – *Drugs in Context*;
   Editor – *BESTMEDICINE*
Dr Jonathan Morrell, GP, Hastings; Medical Editor (Primary Care) –
   Drugs in Context
Dr Michael Schachter, Consultant Physician, St Mary's Hospital
   Paddington; Clinical Pharmacology Editor – *Drugs in Context*

Reader's guide

We acknowledge that some of the medical and scientific terminology used throughout *BESTMEDICINE* will be new to you and will address sometimes challenging concepts. However, rather than abridge the content and risk excluding important information, we have included this Reader's Guide to dissect and explain the contents of *BESTMEDICINE* in order to make it more digestible to the less scientifically minded reader. We recommend that you familiarise yourself with the drug development process, summarised below, before embarking on the Drug Reviews. This brief synopsis clarifies and contextualises many of the specialist terms encountered in the Drug Reviews.

Following this Reader's Guide, you will find that *BESTMEDICINE* is made up of two main sections – a Disease Overview and the Drug Reviews – both of which are evidence-based and as such have been highly referenced. All references are listed at the end of a section. Importantly, the manuscript has been 'peer-reviewed', which means that it has undergone rigorous checks for accuracy both by a practising doctor and a specialist in drug pharmacology. The Disease Overview and Drug Reviews are sandwiched between two opinion pieces, an Editorial, written by a recognised expert in the field, and an Improving Practice article, written by a practising GP with a specialist interest in the disease area. It is important to bear in mind that these authors are addressing their professional colleagues, rather than a 'lay' reader, providing you with a fascinating and unique insight into many of the challenges faced by doctors in the day-to-day practice of medicine.

The Disease Overview, Drug Reviews and Improving Practice sections are all followed by a short commentary by Dr Steve Illiffe entitled Patient Notes. In these sections, Dr Steve Illiffe reiterates some of the key issues raised in rather more 'user-friendly' language.

As mentioned previously, much of the content of *BESTMEDICINE* has been taken directly from *Drugs in Context,* which is written by and for healthcare professionals. Consequently, some of the language used may be difficult for the less scientifically minded reader. To help with this, in addition to the Patient Notes, we have included a comprehensive glossary of those terms underlined in the text. Terms will not be underlined in tables or figures, but the more difficult words will be defined in the Glossary.

Disease overview

The disease overview provides a brief synopsis of the disease, its symptoms, diagnosis and a critique of the currently available treatment options.
- The epidemiology, or incidence and distribution of the disease within a population, is discussed, with particular emphasis on UK-specific data.

- The <u>aetiology</u> section describes the specific causes or origins of the disease, which are usually a result of both genetic and environmental factors. <u>Multifactorial</u> diseases result from more than one causative element. If an individual has a <u>genetic predisposition</u>, they are more susceptible to developing the disease as a result of their genetic make-up.
- The functional changes that accompany a particular syndrome or disease constitute its <u>pathophysiology</u>.
- The management of a disease may be influenced by treatment guidelines, specific directives published by government agencies, professional societies, or by the convening of expert panels. The National Institute for Clinical Excellence (NICE), an independent sector of the NHS comprised of experts in the field of treatment, is one such body.
- The social and economic factors that characterise the influence of the disease, describe its <u>socioeconomic impact</u>. Such factors include the cost to the healthcare provider to treat the disease – in terms of GP consultations, drug costs and the subsequent burden on hospital resources – or the cost to the patient or employer with respect to the number of work days lost as a consequence of ill health.

Drug reviews

☛ *The <u>pharmacokinetics</u> of a drug are of interest to healthcare professionals because it is important for them to understand the action of a drug on the body over a period of time.*

The drug reviews are not intended to address every available treatment for a particular disease. Rather, we focus on the major drugs currently available in the UK for the treatment of the featured disease and evaluate their performance in clinical trials and their safety in clinical practice. The basic <u>pharmacology</u> of the drug – the branch of science that deals with the origin, nature, chemistry, effects and uses of drugs – is discussed initially. This includes a description of the <u>mechanism of action</u> of the drug, the manner in which it exerts its therapeutic effects, and its <u>pharmacokinetics</u> (or the activity of the drug within the body over a period of time). Pharmacokinetics encompasses the <u>absorption</u> of the drug into or across the tissues of the body, its distribution to specific functional areas, its <u>metabolism</u> – the process by which it is broken down within the body into by-products (<u>metabolites</u>) – and ultimately, its removal or <u>excretion</u> from the body. The most frequently used pharmacokinetic terms that are used in the drug review sections of this issue of *BESTMEDICINE* are explained in Table 1.

Whilst the basic <u>pharmacology</u> of a drug is clearly important, the main focus of the drug review is to summarise the drug's performance in controlled clinical trials. Clinical trials examine the effectiveness, or clinical <u>efficacy</u>, of the drug against the disease or condition it was developed to treat, as well as its <u>safety and tolerability</u> – the side-effects associated with the drug and the likelihood that the patient will tolerate treatment. Adherence to drug treatment, or patient compliance, reflects the tendency of patients to comply with the terms of their treatment regimen. Compliance may be affected by treatment-related side-effects or the convenience of drug treatment. The safety of the drug also

Table 1. Key terms.

Term	Definition
Agonist	A drug/substance that has affinity for specific cell receptors thereby triggering a biological response.
Antagonist	A drug/substance that blocks the action of another by binding to a specific cell receptor without eliciting a biological response.
AUC (area under curve)	A plot of the concentration of a drug against the time since initial administration. It is a means of analysing the bioavailability of a drug.
Binding affinity	An attractive force between substances that causes them to enter into and remain in chemical contact.
Bioavailability	The degree and rate at which a drug is absorbed into a living system or is made available at the site of physiological activity.
Clearance	The rate at which the drug is removed from the blood by excretion into the urine through the kidneys.
C_{max}	The maximum concentration of the drug recorded in the blood plasma.
Cytochrome P450 (CYP) system	A group of enzymes responsible for the metabolism of a number of different drugs and substances within the body.
Dose dependency	In which the effect of the drug is proportional to the concentration of drug administered.
Enzyme	A protein produced in the body that catalyses chemical reactions without itself being destroyed or altered. The suffix 'ase' is used when designating an enzyme.
Excretion	The elimination of a waste product (in faeces or urine) from the body.
Half-life ($t_{1/2}$)	The time required for half the original amount of a drug to be eliminated from the body by natural processes.
Inhibitor	A substance that reduces the activity of another substance.
Ligand	Any substance that binds to another and brings about a biological response.
Potency	A measure of the power of a drug to produce the desired effects.
Protein binding	The extent to which a drug attaches to proteins, peptides or enzymes within the body.
Receptor	A molecular structure, usually (but not always) situated on the cell membrane, which mediates the biological response that is associated with a particular drug/substance.
Synergism	A phenomenon in which the combined effects of two drugs are more powerful than when either drug is administered alone.
t_{max}	The time taken to reach C_{max}.
Volume of distribution (V_D)	The total amount of drug in the body divided by its concentration in the blood plasma. Used as a measure of the dispersal of the drug within the body once it has been absorbed.

encompasses its <u>contra-indications</u>, conditions under which the drug should never be prescribed. This may mean avoiding use in special patient populations (e.g. young or elderly patients, or those with co-existing or <u>comorbid</u> conditions, such as liver or kidney disease) or avoiding <u>co-administration</u> with certain other medications.

A brief synopsis of the drug development process is outlined below, in order to clarify and put into context many of the specialist terms encountered throughout the drug reviews.

The drug development process

Launching a new drug is an extremely costly and time-consuming venture. The entire process can cost an estimated £500 million and can take between 10 and 15 years from the initial identification of a potentially useful therapeutic compound in the laboratory to launching the finished product as a treatment for a particular disease (Figure 1). Much of this time is spent fulfilling strict guidelines set out by regulatory authorities, in order to ensure the safety and quality of the end product. As a consequence of this, a drug can fail at any stage of the development process and its development abandoned. Once identified and registered, the new drug can be protected by a patent for 20 years, after which time other companies are free to manufacture and market identical drugs, called generics. Thus, the pharmaceutical company has a finite period of time before patent expiry to recoup the cost of drug development (of both successful drugs and those drugs that do not make it to the marketplace) and return a profit to their shareholders.

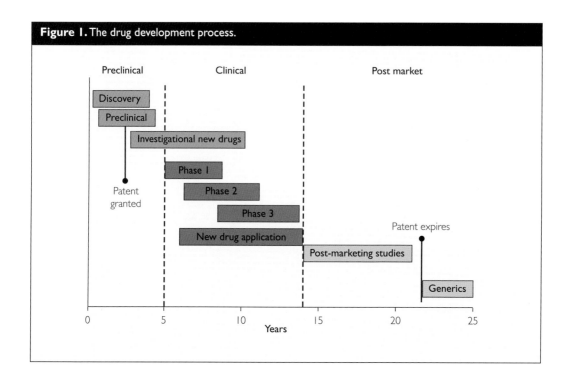

Figure 1. The drug development process.

Potential new drugs are identified by the research and development (R&D) department of the pharmaceutical company. After a candidate drug has been selected for development, it enters a rigorous testing procedure with five distinct phases – preclinical, which takes place in the laboratory, and phases 1, 2, 3 and 4, which involve testing in humans. Approval from the regulatory body is essential before the drug can be marketed and is dependent on the satisfactory completion of all phases of testing. In the UK, the Medicines and Healthcare Products Agency (MHRA) and the European Medicines Evaluation Agency (EMEA) regulate the development process and companies must apply to these organisations for marketing authorisation. Within Europe, the Mutual Recognition Procedure means that the approval of a drug in one country (the Reference Member State), forms the basis for its subsequent approval in other European Union member states. This can make the approval process more efficient and may lead to approval being granted in several European countries at once. Once approval has been granted, the drug will be given a licence detailing the specific disease or conditions it is indicated to treat and the patient groups it may be used in. The drug will be assigned either prescription-only medicine (POM) or over-the counter (OTC) status. POMs can only be obtained following consultation with a doctor, who will actively supervise their use.

Preclinical testing

Preclinical testing is essential before a drug can progress to human clinical trials. It is estimated that only one of every 1000 compounds that enter the preclinical stage continue into human testing (phases 1–4). Preclinical testing, or screening, is for the main-part performed in animals, and every effort is made to use as few animals as possible and to ensure their humane and proper care. Generally, two or more species (one rodent, one non-rodent) are tested, since a drug may affect one species differently from another.

Although a drug will never act in exactly the same way in animals as in humans, animal models are designed to mimic a human disease condition as closely as possible and provide information essential to drug development. *In vitro* experiments – literally meaning 'in glass' – are performed outside the living system in a laboratory setting. *In vivo* experiments are performed in the living cell or organism.

It is during the preclinical phase that the pharmacodynamics of the drug will first be examined. These include its mechanism of action, or the way in which it exerts its therapeutic effects. The drug's pharmacokinetics, toxicology (potentially hazardous or poisonous effects) and the formulation of the drug – the manner in which it is taken (e.g. tablet, injection, liquid) – are also assessed at this point in development.

Phase I

Phase 1 trials are usually conducted in a small group of 10–80 healthy volunteers and further evaluate the biochemical and physiological effects of the drug – its chemical and biological impact within the body. An appropriate dosage range will be established at this point – the maximum and minimum therapeutic concentrations of the drug which are associated with a tolerable number of side-effects (secondary and usually <u>adverse events</u> unrelated to the beneficial effects of the drug). The mechanism of action and pharmacokinetic effects of the drugs are also further explored in this, the first group of human subjects to receive the drug.

Phase 2

If no major problems are revealed during phase 1 development, the drug can progress to phase 2 screening which takes place in 100–300 patients diagnosed with the disease or condition that the drug is designed to treat. At this stage it is important to determine the effectiveness, or <u>efficacy</u>, of the drug. If the drug is no better than <u>placebo</u> then it will not be granted a licence. The side-effect or adverse event profile of the drug is re-examined at this stage, and is particularly pertinent in these patients, who may react more severely to the drug than healthy volunteers. The likelihood and severity of <u>drug interactions</u> is also of great importance in this patient group. Drug interactions – in which the action of one drug interferes with the action of another – can occur if the patient is taking more than one form of medication for the treatment of a <u>comorbid</u> disease or condition. If multiple drugs are administered together, or concomitantly, then the risk of drug interactions is increased.

Phase 3

Phase 3 clinical trials involve between 1000 and 3000 patients diagnosed with the relevant disease or condition. The recruitment of patients and the co-ordination and analysis of the trials is costly, so the pharmaceutical company will not embark on this stage unless they are sufficiently convinced of the therapeutic benefits of their drug. Essentially, phase 3 trials are replications of phase 2 trials but on a larger scale. The duration of the trial depends on the type of drug and the length of time required in order to determine the <u>efficacy</u> of the drug. For example, an antibiotic trial will have a shorter duration than the trial of a drug intended to treat long-term conditions, such as Alzheimer's disease. <u>Acute</u> treatment describes a short-term schedule given over a period of days or weeks, and <u>chronic</u> treatment refers to longer-term treatment schedules, lasting over periods of months or years.

Clinical trials may compare the new drug with an existing drug – a comparative trial – or may simply compare the new drug with no active drug treatment at all – a <u>placebo-controlled</u> trial. The participants who receive a comparator treatment or placebo are termed controls. In placebo-controlled trials, patients are given a placebo – an inert substance with no specific pharmacological activity – in place of the active drug. Patients will be unaware that the substance they are taking is placebo, which will be visually identical to the active treatment. This approach rules out any psychological effects of drug treatment – a patient may perceive that their condition has improved simply through the action of taking a tablet. In order to be considered clinically effective, the experimental drug must produce better results than the placebo.

The clinical trial should be designed in such a way as to limit the degree of bias it carries. The blinding of the trial is one means of eliminating bias. Double-blind trials, in which neither the doctor nor the patient knows which is the real drug and which is the placebo or comparator drug, are the most informative. In single-blind trials, only the patient is unaware of what they are taking, and in open-label trials, all participants are aware of treatment allocation. Conducting the trial across a number of clinics or hospitals, either abroad or in the same country (multicentre trials), further eliminates bias, as does randomisation, the random allocation of patients to treatment groups. At the start of the study, the baseline characteristics of the study population are recorded and are used as a starting point for all subsequent comparisons.

☛ *Someone is always aware of who is taking what in a clinical trial. Whilst neither a doctor nor a patient may be aware of their treatment in a double-blind trial, there is a secure coding system, known only to the investigator, which contains the various treatment allocations.*

Efficacy is commonly measured by means of primary and secondary endpoints. Endpoints mark a recognised stage in the disease process and are used to compare the outcome in different treatment arms of clinical trials. The endpoint of one trial may be a marker of improvement or recovery whereas another trial may use the deterioration of the patient (morbidity) or death (mortality) to signify the end of the trial. Either way, endpoints represent valid criteria by which to compare treatments. On a similar note, surrogate markers are laboratory measurements of biological activity within the body that provide an indirect measure of the effect of treatment on disease state (e.g. blood pressure and cholesterol levels).

Statistical analysis allows the investigator to draw rational conclusions from clinical trials regarding the effectiveness of their drug. If the patient data generated during the course of a clinical trial are statistically significant, then there is a high probability that the given result, be it an improvement or a decline in the health of the patient, is due to a specific effect of drug treatment, rather than a chance occurrence. The data are put through a number of mathematical procedures that ultimately produce a *p*-value. This value reflects the probability that the result occurred by chance. For example, if the *p*-value is less than or equal to 0.05, the result is usually considered to be statistically significant. Such a *p*-value indicates that there is a 95% probability that the result did not occur by chance. The smaller the *p*-value, the more significant the result. When quoting clinical findings, the *p*-value is often given in brackets in order to emphasise the importance of the finding.

Once a drug has progressed through the key stages of development and demonstrated clear efficacy with an acceptable safety profile, the data are collated and the pharmaceutical company will then submit a licence application to the regulatory authorities – a new drug application (NDA).

Phase 4 (Post-marketing studies)

Phase 4 testing takes place after the drug has been marketed and involves large numbers of patients, sometimes including those groups that may have previously been excluded from clinical trials (e.g. pregnant women and elderly or young patients). These trials are usually <u>open-label</u>, so the patient is aware of what they are taking, without control groups. They provide valuable information regarding the tolerability of the drug, and may reveal any long-term <u>adverse events</u> associated with treatment. Post-marketing surveillance continues throughout the life-span of the drug, and constantly monitors the safety, usage and performance. Doctors are advised to inform the MHRA and the Committee on Safety of Medicines (CSM) of any adverse events they encounter.

Editorial

Professor Susan M Benbow
Professor of Mental Health and Ageing
University of Wolverhampton
Consultant Old Age Psychiatrist
Wolverhampton City Primary Care Trust

The treatment of Alzheimer's disease has changed enormously over the last 10 years. The first antidementia drug licensed for use in the United Kingdom (donepezil [Aricept®]), an <u>acetylcholinesterase inhibitor</u>, was introduced in 1997 and has since been joined by others including rivastigmine (Exelon®) and galantamine (Reminyl®). Initially, purchasing authorities were reluctant to budget for the use of these drugs, ostensibly because of concern about the potential cost of treating large numbers of people with memory problems presumed due to Alzheimer's disease, and because improvements demonstrated in clinical trials were deemed not to satisfy the demands of stringent reviewers. In reality, the reluctance to fund probably resulted from overtly ageist attitudes: are older adults with progressive <u>cognitive</u> impairment 'worth' the expenditure in a cash-limited health service; are short-term improvements in symptoms 'worth' the expenditure in resources?

The National Institute for Clinical Excellence (NICE) published guidance on the use of acetylcholinesterase inhibitors in January 2001. This guidance was under review as this issue of *BESTMEDICINE* went to press and will include guidance on memantine (Ebixa®), which was introduced in 2002. Randomised controlled trials of the acetylcholinesterase inhibitors had shown statistically significant improvements in cognitive function above <u>baseline</u> values for all three drugs, but treatment was generally assessed over relatively short periods and the effect size was 'modest'. Evidence of improvement in quality of life was dismissed by NICE in 2001 as 'mixed' and cost-effectiveness had not been established. The 2001 NICE guidance recommended drug treatment as 'one component' in the management of Alzheimer's disease, with a Mini-Mental State Examination (MMSE) (see Disease Overview p. 6) score of 12 given as the cut off for treatment. This guidance also required specialists to make the diagnosis of Alzheimer's disease and to initiate treatment, and set out conditions for assessing people prior to initiation of therapy and for reviewing people on treatment. The Older People's National Service Framework (OP NSF) reiterated these requirements and listed consideration of antidementia drug treatment as one of the reasons for referring people on to specialist older adults' mental health services.

Many old-age psychiatry services developed memory clinics to support antidementia drug treatment. Most are hospital based and were listed as a secondary care component of the service model for older people's mental health services set out in the OP NSF.

☛ *Remember that the author of this Editorial is addressing her healthcare professional colleagues rather than the 'lay' reader. This provides a fascinating insight into many of the challenges faced by doctors in the day-to-day practice of medicine (see Reader's Guide).*

☛ *The MMSE is a quantative measure of cognitive status in adults.*

However, GPs are beginning to question the need for initiation and monitoring of antidementia drugs within secondary care. Could GPs take a lead using agreed shared care protocols, could memory clinics move out of secondary care into primary care? The Audit Commission report *Forget Me Not*, published in 2000, stated that fewer than half of GPs felt that they had sufficient training to diagnose and manage <u>dementia</u>, and only just over half agreed that it is important to look for early signs of dementia and to make an early diagnosis. Fewer than half were using protocols at that time to assist in the diagnosis and management of dementia. However, services have moved on since then. For example, one of the milestones in Standard 7 of the OP NSF was that by April 2004 every general practice should be using a protocol agreed with local specialist health and social services for the diagnosis, care and treatment of people with dementia.

Currently there are still concerns that the prescribing of antidementia drugs is not equitable across the country. Ageist inequities are becoming less tenable as carers and people with dementia themselves become more vocal about their needs. For the future the move towards greater GP involvement in antidementia drug prescribing is likely to become stronger, and memory clinics may move towards primary care. Ongoing research is likely to clarify the role of drug treatment for Alzheimer's disease, and to extend drug treatments to a broader diagnostic group (some evidence already supports <u>efficacy</u> in <u>Lewy Body</u> dementia and mixed <u>vascular</u>/Alzheimer's disease) and to people with more severe <u>cognitive</u> impairments. At the same time the need for psychological and social treatments will also become more sharply defined, whilst future generations of people with dementia and their families will be less prepared to accept ageist attitudes to care.

Editor's note: This editorial by Professor Benbow first appeared in *Drugs in Context*, which was published in April 2004. As Professor Benbow highlights, guidance from the National Institute for Clinical Excellence (NICE) on the use of donepezil, galantamine, memantine and rivastigmine was undergoing review when this issue of *Drugs in Context* was published. However, as this edition of *BESTMEDICINE* goes to press (March 2005), the institute has issued preliminary guidance on the use of these drugs in the NHS, which reverses its original guidance and recommends against the use of these drugs for new patients. Whilst the institute acknowledges that each drug offers clinically relevant benefits, both in controlled clinical trials and in real clinical practice, it argues that economic evaluations puts these drugs outside the range of cost-effectiveness that NICE considers acceptable for the NHS. However, it is important to remember that this is preliminary guidance, and is subject to further consultation and review involving a number of parties, including patient support groups and the manufacturers of the drugs. Indeed, as we go to press, the opposition to this preliminary guidance has gathered pace, with the UK Health Minister, Stephen Ladyman, urging NICE to reconsider the wider implications of not approving the drugs' use, in particular the benefits and costs to carers as well as patients. Hundreds of people have also called for an end to dementia discrimination at a mass lobby of parliament organised by the Alzheimer's Society.

The final recommendation from NICE on the use of these drugs in Alzheimer's disease is not expected to be published until October 2005. In the intervening period, we will keep readers abreast of developments through our website (*www.bestmedicine.com*), and as soon as the final guidance from NICE is announced, we will publish a second edition of *BESTMEDICINE Alzheimer's Disease*, which will clarify what this guidance means for patients and their families. In the meantime, we hope that the information that you find in this book will be valuable when discussing long-term care with healthcare professionals.

I. Disease overview – Alzheimer's disease

Dr Richard Clark
CSF Medical Communications Ltd

Summary

Alzheimer's disease is a progressive <u>neurodegenerative</u> disorder,
resulting in the syndrome of Alzheimer's <u>dementia</u>. The most
common form of dementia, Alzheimer's accounts for about 65% of
all dementias and can be either familial or <u>sporadic</u> in nature.
Familial Alzheimer's disease is relatively uncommon and
predominantly affects patients under the age of 65 years, whereas
the sporadic form is rare in people under 60 years of age, yet
affects one person in 20 aged over 65 years and one person in five
over 80 years of age. Symptoms of Alzheimer's disease are revealed
gradually such that a close family member rather than the sufferers
themselves are often first to notice a change in personality. In fact,
the early symptoms of Alzheimer's disease are frequently mistaken
for signs of the normal ageing process or other conditions such as
depression. As the disease progresses, patients experience
increased memory loss such that they will eventually fail to
recognise close family and friends. They also need more and more
help to perform normal daily tasks, and eventually become totally
dependent on others for nursing care. The economic burden on
society is huge as long-term nursing care is costly. Alzheimer's
disease is a life-shortening illness, with death usually occurring
within 5–10 years of diagnosis. As the disease itself is irreversible,
treatments for Alzheimer's disease address <u>cognitive</u> and
behavioural symptoms. Non-pharmacological treatments involve
the manipulation of the patient's environment and the introduction
of structured behaviours and activities. Most current
pharmacological treatments are focused on reducing the
<u>cholinergic</u> deficit that characterises Alzheimer's disease (e.g. by
using <u>cholinesterase inhibitors</u>). Drugs of this class, of which there
are three approved treatments currently available for mild or

moderate dementia, have shown efficacy in stabilising – and in some patients improving – the decline in cognitive function, delaying the need for placement in a nursing home and improving disruptive behaviours. Memantine – an N-methyl-D-aspartate (NMDA) antagonist – is available to treat moderate-to-severe Alzheimer's disease – and prevents the pathological activation of the NMDA receptor.

The burden and impact of Alzheimer's disease

Alzheimer's disease is a progressive neurodegenerative disorder, causing the syndrome of Alzheimer's dementia (Table 1).[1] Alzheimer's disease is defined clinically by a gradual decline in memory, plus at least one other area of higher intellectual function.[2] The domains affected are cognition (e.g. memory loss, impaired judgement and disorientation), daily functioning (e.g. difficulty in performing normal day-to-day activities, such as washing/bathing, dressing) and behaviour (e.g. changes in mood, personality and loss of initiative) (Table 2).[2,3] Onset may occur from the age of 45, but typically occurs after 65 years.[4] The early onset of the disease, before 65 years of age, is strongly associated with familial inheritance. It is important, particularly in terms of treatment approaches, to distinguish Alzheimer's disease from other common forms of dementia, which include vascular, Lewy body and fronto-temporal dementias, including Pick's disease (Figure 1).[5] Some patients may present with a combination of dementia-related diseases.

In the UK, the prevalence of dementia is about 1%, and there are over 775,000 cases of dementia.

Dementia is a common disorder, affecting approximately 18 million people worldwide, with figures predicted to nearly double to 34 million by 2025 in line with shifting population demographics.[6] In the UK, the prevalence of dementia is about 1%, and there are currently over 775,000 cases of dementia.[5,7] By 2010 there will be about 840,000 people with dementia in the UK, a figure that is expected to rise to over 1.5 million cases by 2050.[5]

Table 1. Definitions of dementia, Alzheimer's dementia and Alzheimer's disease.[1]

Term	Definition
Alzheimer's disease	Progressive neurodegeneration with distinctive histopathology
Alzheimer's dementia	The symptoms of Alzheimer's disease, marked by a gradual decline in memory, plus at least one other area of higher intellectual function
Dementia	Chronic or persistent disorder of the mental processes marked by memory disorders, personality changes, impaired reasoning etc. due to injury or brain disease, the most common form of which is Alzheimer's dementia

Table 2. The domains of function and symptoms of Alzheimer's disease.[2,3]

Domains affected	Symptoms
Cognition	Memory loss
	Language problems
	Disorientation
	Impaired judgement
	Misplacing items
Function	Difficulties in performing day-to-day activities:
	• instrumental activities of daily living
	• basic activities of daily living
	Difficulties in performing complex tasks
Behaviour	Changes in mood or behaviour:
	• aggression, agitation, depression
	Changes in personality
	Loss of initiative

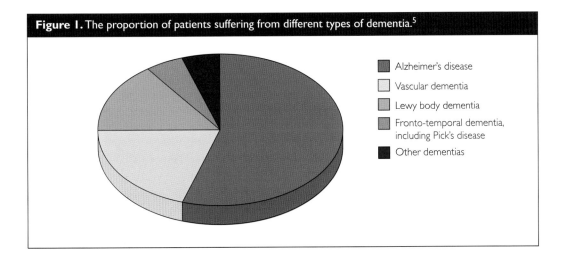

Figure 1. The proportion of patients suffering from different types of dementia.[5]

- Alzheimer's disease
- Vascular dementia
- Lewy body dementia
- Fronto-temporal dementia, including Pick's disease
- Other dementias

Dementia is comparatively rare in people under 60 years of age, but its prevalence increases sharply with advancing age amongst those in their 70s and 80s (Figure 2).[8,9] Dementia affects one person in 20 aged over 65 years and one person in five over 80 years of age.[5] Alzheimer's disease is the most common type of dementia, accounting for over half of all cases. Overall, most studies show that Alzheimer's disease is as common in men as in women, though some evidence suggests a slightly higher prevalence rate may occur amongst women.[6,9]

The Audit Commission has estimated that dementia costs the UK £6.1 billion annually (at 1998–99 prices), with £3.3 billion as direct spend by the NHS and social services.[10,11] Patients with dementia are about four-times more likely than those without dementia to require institutionalised care, and institutionalisation is responsible for the largest proportion of

> Alzheimer's disease is the most common type of dementia, accounting for over half of all cases.

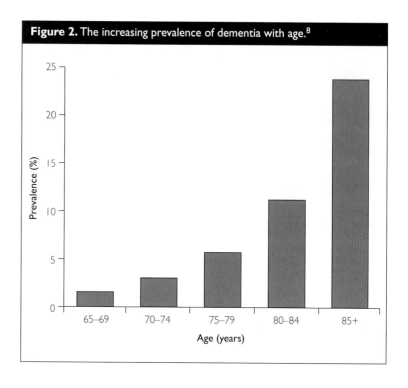

Figure 2. The increasing prevalence of dementia with age.[8]

costs.[12] The pharmacological treatment of Alzheimer's disease with cholinesterase inhibitors can reduce the economic burden of the disease by delaying patients' progression to the nursing home, as reported by a study of tacrine[a], rivastigmine and donepezil.[13] Thus, although the annual cost to the NHS of prescribing a <u>cholinesterase inhibitor</u> for Alzheimer's disease is estimated at about £800–1200 per patient, a delay of 12 weeks in nursing home placement would accrue a saving of £4500 per patient.[11,14] The cost of treating Alzheimer's disease increases with the severity of the disease state, as evidenced by the increased costs associated with increments in the <u>Neuropsychiatric Inventory (NPI) scale</u>.[15] Patients with advanced disease are more expensive to treat in terms of their use of hospital resources, the number of physician consultations and the caregiver burden.[16]

Diagnosis and measuring dementia

The symptoms of Alzheimer's disease start gradually and as patients are generally unaware of the gradual deterioration in their memory, it is common for a family member or close friend to recognise the problem.[17] It is important that the emergence of memory and <u>cognitive</u> deficits, as indicators of Alzheimer's disease, are differentiated from other possible causes of cognitive decline, which may include old age, depression, <u>hypercalcaemia</u> and side-effects from concomitant medications. The term mild cognitive impairment (MCI) was proposed to describe the

> As patients are generally unaware of the gradual deterioration in their memory it is common for a family member or close friend to recognise the problem.

[a]Tacrine is not currently licensed in the UK.

transitional state between normal cognition and Alzheimer's disease. Conventionally defined MCI has reasonable predictive value and specificity for Alzheimer's disease with an estimated 8% of MCI patients converting annually.[18] However, not all patients with MCI and the worsening of <u>episodic memory</u> will convert to Alzheimer's disease.[19]

Since approximately 74% of <u>dementia</u> patients will first present to a doctor in a primary-care setting, GPs in particular, should be aware of signs that are indicative of Alzheimer's disease.[20] The following points are worthwhile of consideration during a consultation.

- Although a patient may not look ill, has a relative or close friend noticed a change in their personality or memory impairment?
- Does the patient have a tendency to look at an accompanying relative or friend when asked a question?
- Does the patient have difficulty recalling the current date?
- Is the patient hesitant in their use of language?
- Do they have a tendency to minimalise/rationalise symptoms?

Prior to referral to a specialist, patients with suspected Alzheimer's disease should undergo routine blood tests, including:

- a full blood count for <u>macrocytic anaemia</u>, suggesting vitamin B_{12}/folate deficiency (or an excessive consumption of alcohol)
- thyroid function tests to exclude hypothyroidism
- a <u>fasting blood glucose test</u>
- a <u>serum calcium test</u>.[4]

Importantly, there is an average delay of 4 months from the first onset of noticeable Alzheimer's disease to the first appointment with a doctor, and a 1-year delay from noticing the first symptoms to diagnosis.[20] This emphasises the importance of the early initiation of treatment for Alzheimer's disease in order to obtain maximum therapeutic benefit (e.g. delaying the progression of Alzheimer's disease and increasing the length of time prior to nursing home placement).[20]

Clinical assessment using rating scales and other assessment tools remains the cornerstone of the diagnostic approach to Alzheimer's disease, although concerns as to the validity and relevance of such scales to the patient population have been voiced. The increased use of <u>positron emission tomography (PET)</u> and <u>magnetic resonance imaging (MRI)</u> to identify changes in glucose <u>metabolism</u> and <u>brain atrophy</u> together with the analysis of <u>biomarkers</u> in <u>cerebrospinal fluid</u> and <u>blood serum</u> (e.g. β-amyloid, total and <u>phosphotau protein</u>) may improve the sensitivity and specificity of diagnosis in the future.

The International statistical classification of diseases and related health problems (ICD-10) outlines criteria for a formal diagnosis of Alzheimer's disease.[1]

(1) The presence of dementia:

- disturbance of <u>higher cortical</u> functions including memory, thinking, orientation, comprehension, calculation, learning capacity, language and judgement
- consciousness is not clouded

> There is an average delay of 1 year from noticing the first symptoms of Alzheimer's disease to diagnosis.

- impairments of <u>cognitive</u> function are commonly accompanied and occasionally preceded by deterioration in emotional control, social behaviour or motivation
- interference with personal activities of daily living such as washing, dressing, eating, personal hygiene, excretory and toilet activities may occur.

(2) Insidious onset with slow deterioration.

(3) Absence of clinical evidence, or findings from special investigations, that the mental state may be due to other systemic or brain disease which can induce <u>dementia</u> (e.g. hypothyroidism, <u>hypercalcaemia</u>, <u>vitamin B$_{12}$ deficiency</u>, <u>niacin deficiency</u>, <u>neurosyphilis</u>, <u>normal pressure hydrocephalus</u> or <u>subdural haematoma</u>).

(4) Absence of a sudden, <u>apoplectic</u> onset, or of neurological signs of focal damage such as <u>hemiparesis</u>, sensory loss, visual field defects and incoordination occurring early in the illness (although these phenomena may be superimposed later).[1]

A diagnosis of Alzheimer's disease can also be made using criteria set out by the National Institute for Neurological and Communicative Disorders and Stroke – Alzheimer's Disease and Related Disorders Association (NINDS ADRDA), which emphasises memory loss as the main feature to distinguish Alzheimer's disease from other forms of dementia. The Diagnostic and Statistical Manual of Mental Disorders (DSM-IV) defines Alzheimer's disease by assessing the severity of cognitive and non-cognitive impairment and classifies Alzheimer's disease according to the age of onset of symptoms and the presence or absence of behavioural disturbances.

☞ *The MMSE is a quantative measure of cognitive status in adults.*

The most widely used test for screening patients in whom dementia is suspected is the Mini-Mental Status Examination (MMSE).[17] However, the MMSE is relatively insensitive in patients with severe dementia, for whom the Severe Impairment Battery (SIB), which evaluates cognitive aptitudes and other skills, is more appropriate. The MMSE has a maximum (best) score of 30, and can be used to grade Alzheimer's disease:

- mild – MMSE score 21–26
- moderate – MMSE score 12–20
- moderately severe – MMSE score 10–11
- severe – MMSE score of nine or less.[14]

Of the components of the MMSE, the clock-drawing test – used as a <u>cognitive</u> screening instrument – is the most useful and simplistic. Commonly, the fourth quadrant of the clock shows the greatest sensitivity for dementia. Although the MMSE is a good test of cognitive function, it takes up to 10 minutes to complete and so does not fit easily into a standard primary-care consultation. In contrast, the Abbreviated Mental Test Score (AMTS) consists of 10 questions and can be completed during a standard GP consultation (Figure 3).

Figure 3. The Abbreviated Mental Test Score (AMTS).

Each correctly answered
question scores one point

1. Age ☐

2. Time to nearest hour ☐

3. An address – for example 42 West Street – to be repeated ☐
    by the patient at the end of the test

4. Year ☐

5. Name of hospital, residential institution or home address, ☐
    depending on where the patient is situated

6. Recognition of two persons – for example, doctor, nurse, home help etc. ☐

7. Date of birth ☐

8. Year First World War started ☐

9. Name of present monarch ☐

10. Count backwards from 20 to 1 ☐

Total score _____

(A score of less than six is suggestive of dementia.)

Course, symptoms and prognosis

As Alzheimer's disease is progressive, the structure and chemistry of the
brain become increasingly altered over time. As a consequence of these
changes, Alzheimer's disease is usually considered as three stages – early,
middle and late. However, in some individuals certain symptoms may
appear earlier, later or not at all, and various stages may overlap.[5] The
behavioural and psychological symptoms of dementia (BPSD) can occur
and disappear during the course of illness, with different symptoms
associated with different stages of the disease. For example, depression
and anxiety are more prevalent in early Alzheimer's disease and

psychosis, agitation and aggression commonly present later on. Guidelines for the management of BPSD have been published by the Scottish Intercollegiate Guidelines Network (*www.sign.ac.uk*) and the International Psychogeriatric Association.[21]

Early stage

Alzheimer's disease tends to begin gradually, so the early symptoms may go unrecognised, frequently being mistaken as normal signs of ageing. Typical symptoms include:
- loss of short-term memory, forgetting recent conversations or events
- decreased judgement, finding decisions harder to make, inability to manage complex tasks (e.g. financial decisions)
- loss of interest in other people or activities
- lack of initiative and becoming slower to grasp new ideas.[5,17]

> Alzheimer's disease tends to begin gradually, so the early symptoms may go unrecognised, frequently being mistaken as normal signs of ageing.

Middle stage

Symptoms become more marked as Alzheimer's disease progresses, and as a consequence patients need increased help with their daily tasks, such as eating, washing and dressing. Typical symptoms include:
- increasing decline in short-term memory leading to forgetfulness, with patients being unable to recognise close friends or family, and often repeating the same phrase many times
- becoming easily upset, angry or aggressive; patients may also become very clinging
- wandering off, becoming lost, and becoming confused about where they are
- difficulty or inability to dress, undress and poor attention to personal hygiene
- behaving in an inappropriate manner (e.g. going outside in nightclothes)
- experiencing paranoid ideas and hallucinations.[5,17]

Specific staging scales can be used to assess the severity of Alzheimer's disease progression and, of these, the Functional Assessment Staging (FAST) system and the Clinical Dementia Rating (CDR) are the most reliable.

> Loss of memory may be close to complete, such that the patient does not recognise familiar objects or surroundings or closest family members, though flashes of recognition can occur.

Late stage

At this stage, patients require a great deal of help and gradually become totally dependent on others for nursing care. Loss of memory may be close to complete, such that they do not recognise familiar objects or surroundings or closest family members, though flashes of recognition can occur. Other symptoms include:
- increasing frailty, shuffling or unsteady gait, eventually becoming confined to bed and/or a wheelchair
- losing control of bladder and bowel functions

- inability to eat unaided
- considerable weight loss
- progressive loss of speech, though they may cry out occasionally or repeat a few words.[5,17]

Dementia can progress for up to 10 years and is a life-shortening illness, though another condition or illness such as <u>bronchopneumonia</u>, may trigger death and be listed as the cause of fatality on the death certificate.[5] Death usually occurs within 5–10 years of diagnosis.[22] As patients' mobility is affected, this can contribute to a decline in physical health and <u>cardiovascular disease</u>; they can be less likely to cope with infections and more likely to die of a <u>pulmonary embolism</u> or a <u>myocardial infarction</u>.[5] However, in some people no specific cause of death is found other than dementia, and therefore it can be listed as sole or main cause of death, or a contributory factor.[5] In England and Wales the <u>mortality</u> rates reported for Alzheimer's disease have increased greatly from 1979 to 1996 (from about 1 to 20 per 100,000 aged over 65 years; Figure 4).[23] However, senile dementia still remains three-times more common than Alzheimer's disease as the underlying cause of death reported on death certificates. Given its greater prevalence, many cases of Alzheimer's disease are thus being misclassified at death as senile <u>dementia</u>.

> Death usually occurs within 5–10 years of diagnosis.

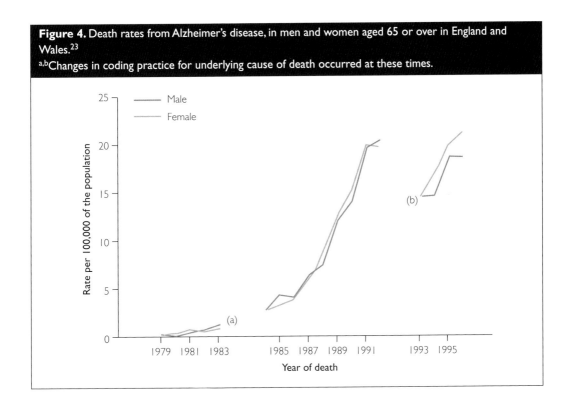

Figure 4. Death rates from Alzheimer's disease, in men and women aged 65 or over in England and Wales.[23]
[a,b]Changes in coding practice for underlying cause of death occurred at these times.

Pathology and aetiology

The aetiology of Alzheimer's disease is unknown.[11] Amyloid plaques and neurofibrillary tangles are commonly associated with Alzheimer's disease and are probably related to the cause, development and course of the disease. However, these pathological markers are not exclusive to Alzheimer's disease and may occur in other dementias and as a result of the normal ageing process.

Amyloid plaques are composed of β-amyloid polypeptides, and seem to form as a result of disorders in processing β-amyloid and its precursor protein, APP, for which a combination of genetic predisposition and environmental factors are probably responsible.[24] Subclinical ischaemia represents one such environmental factor, particularly as patients with hypertension and elevated cholesterol tend to be at increased risk of developing Alzheimer's disease.[25] In reaction to amyloid, the microglia are stimulated to intense metabolic activity, and the resulting increase in cellular respiration consumes oxygen and generates highly reactive oxygen-containing free radicals.[12] These can cause oxidative damage to the cell, the by-products of which can cause further microglial activation that is associated with neurodegeneration.

> When neurones die in Alzheimer's disease neurofibrillary tangles are found between surviving neurones, and have thus been likened to neuronal 'gravestones'.

Neurofibrillary tangles are essentially biochemical modifications of the natural neuronal cytoskeleton; when neurones die in Alzheimer's disease neurofibrillary tangles are found between surviving neurones, and have thus been likened to neuronal 'gravestones'.[12] A key component of the tangles is derived from a naturally occurring microtubule protein, tau. In Alzheimer's disease tau is hyperphosphorylated or glycated, and thus much more likely to form tangles.[12] It is unclear whether these tangles are linked to senile plaque formation, but their ultimate effect is to compromise microtubular function, leading to the eventual destruction of neurones.[24]

In addition to the actions of β-amyloid, oxidative neuronal damage and pathobiology of tau proteins' conversion to neurofibrillary tangles, neurotransmitter depletion also plays a central role in Alzheimer's disease.[26] Alzheimer's disease is associated with deficits in acetylcholine, noradrenaline, serotonin and glutamate. The cognitive decline associated with Alzheimer's disease is primarily attributed to the loss of cholinergic neurons in the cortex and hippocampus, and cholinergic deficiencies are also implicated in the formation of amyloid plaques and neurofibrillary tangles.[22,27] Abnormalities of the cholinergic system, including the upregulation of the cholineacetyltransferase enzyme, ChAT, and abnormal neuronal sprouting, characterise early disease progression.

> Cholinergic deficits are correlated with the cognitive decline and behavioural symptoms associated with Alzheimer's disease.

Cholinergic deficits are also correlated with the cognitive decline and behavioural symptoms associated with Alzheimer's disease.[28,29]

In light of the accumulated evidence for the role of a cholinergic deficit in Alzheimer's disease, early symptomatic treatment focuses on the restoration of this function. Acetylcholinesterase inhibitors are approved in the UK for the treatment of mild-to-moderate Alzheimer's disease. Individual members of this pharmacological class also exert non-cholinergic actions which may be relevant to their clinical efficacy, such as:

- binding to the <u>allosteric activator</u> site on <u>nicotinic receptors</u>
- increasing non-cholinergic neurotransmitter release
- inhibiting β-amyloid toxicity
- increasing <u>soluble β-amyloid precursor protein release</u>
- modulating the effects of <u>oestrogens</u>.[30]

Risk factors

There are multiple risk factors for Alzheimer's disease. However, there is some controversy over which elements are true risk factors, though the strongest evidence is for increased age (the disease is rare in those younger than 60 years but increases to about 24% of those aged ≥85 years).[31] Other risk factors include:

- a family history of <u>dementia</u> (children, brothers or sisters of a person with Alzheimer's disease are three- or four-times more likely to develop this disease than someone with no affected relatives)
- mutations of genes for <u>familial</u> Alzheimer's disease (e.g. <u>presenilin</u> 1 and 2, amyloid prescursor protein)
- mutations of susceptibility genes for <u>sporadic</u> Alzheimer's disease (e.g. apolipoprotein E4)
- low educational attainment (Alzheimer's disease is less common in those with higher levels of education)
- long-standing alcohol abuse
- <u>cardiovascular disease</u> and risk factors
- the presence of Down syndrome; those who survive to late adulthood develop Alzheimer's disease, probably due to genetic disturbances (90% of people with Down syndrome have <u>amyloid plaques</u>, <u>neurofibrillary tangles</u> and <u>cholinergic</u> deficits at 30 years of age; 75% exhibit dementia by the age of 60 years).[17,31–35]

Older people with depression may also be at an increased risk of developing Alzheimer's disease, but whether depression is simply an early symptom or increases susceptibility through another mechanism remains to be determined.[36]

Treatment

Treatments for Alzheimer's disease address <u>cognitive</u> and behavioural symptoms as the disease itself is, at present, irreversible. Traditional approaches involving the manipulation of the patient's environment and the introduction of structured behaviours and activities may be useful.[2] Support group activities, hobbies and outings may reduce anger, depression and anxiety in patients with mild Alzheimer's disease.[2] As the disease progresses changes to patients' immediate surroundings, including the alteration and simplification of living spaces, may also be helpful.[2,3] There are limited data to suggest that some preventative measures may be effective in Alzheimer's disease, such as eating oily fish at least once a week or increasing the intake of <u>antioxidants</u> from food (e.g. vitamins C and E).[37–40]

The <u>cholinesterase</u> <u>inhibitors</u> donepezil, galantamine and rivastigmine are the current recommended standard of care for the treatment of mild-to- moderately severe Alzheimer's disease.

To date, pharmacological treatments have addressed the cholinergic deficit associated with Alzheimer's disease, usually by preventing its breakdown. The <u>cholinesterase inhibitors</u> donepezil, galantamine and rivastigmine are the current recommended standard of care for the treatment of mild-to-moderately severe Alzheimer's disease.[41] Treatment with cholinesterase inhibitors can stabilise and in some cases improve cognition and disruptive behaviour. Furthermore, nursing home placement has been shown to be delayed by almost 2 years following donepezil treatment in comparison with <u>placebo</u>.[35] The NMDA-receptor antagonist, memantine, is also indicated for moderately severe-to-severe Alzheimer's disease. Memantine allows the physiological activation of NMDA receptors during memory formation but blocks the effects of the toxic accumulation of <u>glutamate</u> that may be responsible for neuronal dysfunction.[42,43] However, there is a relative paucity of published data for the use of memantine in comparison with that for the <u>cholinesterase inhibitors</u>. Some guidelines (excluding the National Institute for Clinical Excellence [NICE] UK guidelines) still recommend the use of vitamin E for treating Alzheimer's disease. Vitamin E has been shown to delay patients' disability, placement in a nursing home, but does not improve <u>cognitive</u> deficits.[24,44]

The treatment of common concurrent disorders such as depression should also be undertaken, as these can add to patients' burden of disability.[17] In these cases a <u>selective serotonin reuptake inhibitor</u> is normally given as first-line treatment. Typical antipsychotic compounds are generally avoided, as they are not only more likely to induce <u>extrapyramidal</u> side-effects, but also because their anticholinergic effects may add to the confusion, restlessness, agitation and <u>akathisia</u> experienced by some patients with Alzheimer's disease.[17]

Key points

- Alzheimer's disease is defined clinically by a gradual decline in memory, plus a reduction in at least one other area of higher intellectual function (i.e. cognition, daily functioning and behaviour).

- In the UK, the prevalence of dementia is about 1%, and there are currently over 775,000 cases of <u>dementia</u>. Its prevalence increases sharply with advancing age amongst those in their 70s and 80s.

- Dementia costs the UK £6.1 billion a year, although the costs of effective treatment need to be offset against savings accrued in delaying the requirement for nursing care.

- Risk factors for Alzheimer's disease include a family history of dementia, mutations in specific genes, mutations in susceptibility genes, low educational attainment, <u>cardiovascular disease</u> and risk factors, long-standing alcohol abuse and Down syndrome.

- The development of amyloid plaques and <u>neurofibrillary tangles</u> in the brains of patients with Alzheimer's disease are probably related to the cause, development and course of the disease.

- The symptoms of Alzheimer's disease start gradually, so patients are often unaware of their own health problems.

- Despite the difficulty in assessing treatment benefit in patients who are chronically declining, symptoms of Alzheimer's disease can be ameliorated by pharmacological intervention.

- Early treatment is vital in order to achieve maximum clinical benefit to the patient.

- The manipulation of the patient's environment and the introduction of structured behaviours and activities can help to address their behavioural and psychological symptoms.

- Cholinesterase inhibitors (donepezil, galantamine and rivastigmine) are the current recommended standard of care for the treatment of mild-to-moderately severe Alzheimer's disease, whilst the NMDA-receptor antagonist, memantine, is licensed for moderately severe-to-severe disease.

Any reference made to guidance from the National Institute of Clinical Excellence (NICE) in the preceding section relates to guidelines published in 2001. As we go to press (March 2005), NICE has issued preliminary guidance that is currently under review and will be finalised and published later in 2005 (see Editor's note Pages xx and 127).

References

A list of the published evidence which has been reviewed in compiling the preceding section of *BESTMEDICINE.*

1 *International Statistical Classification of Diseases and Related Health Problems, tenth revision (ICD-10).* Geneva: World Health Organization, 1992.

2 Grossberg GT. The ABC of Alzheimer's disease: behavioral symptoms and their treatment. *Int Psychogeriatr* 2002; **14(Suppl 1)**: 27–49.

3 Potkin SG. The ABC of Alzheimer's disease: ADL and improving day-to-day functioning of patients. *Int Psychogeriatr* 2002; **14(Suppl 1)**: 7–26.

4 Dementia: diagnosis and management in primary care. *http://www.alzheimers.org.uk*

5 Alzheimer's Society website. *http://www.alzheimers.org.uk*

6 Alzheimer's Disease International website. *http://www.alz.co.uk*

7 World Health Organization guide to mental and neurological health in primary care. 2nd edition. London: Royal Society of Medicine Press, 2004.

8 Prince M, Jorm A. Alzheimer's Disease International website. Factsheet 3. The prevalence of dementia. *http://www.alz.co.uk*

9 Jorm AF, Korten AE, Henderson AS. The prevalence of dementia: a quantitative integration of the literature. *Acta Psychiatr Scand* 1987; **76**: 465–79.

10 Audit Commission. *Forget me not.* Portsmouth: Holbrooks, 2000.

11 O'Brien JT, Ballard CG. Drugs for Alzheimer's disease. *BMJ* 2001; **323**: 123–4.

12 Whalley L, Breitner J. *Dementia.* Oxford: Oxford Health Press, 2002.

13 Lopez O, Becker J, Wisniewski S *et al.* Cholinesterase inhibitor treatment alters the natural history of Alzheimer's disease. *J Neurol Neurosurg Psychiatry* 2002; **72**: 310–14.

14 National Institute for Clinical Excellence. Guidance on the use of donepezil, rivastigmine and galantamine for the treatment of Alzheimer's disease. Technology Appraisal Guideline No.19 (2001). *www.nice.org.uk*

15 Murman D, Chen Q, Powell M *et al.* The incremental direct costs associated with behavioral symptoms in AD. *Neurology* 2002; **59**: 1721–9.

16 Small G, McDonnell D, Brooks R, Papadopoulos G. The impact of symptom severity on the cost of Alzheimer's disease. *J Am Geriatr Soc* 2002; **50**: 321–7.

17 Ahmed MB. Alzheimer's disease: recent advances in etiology, diagnosis, and management. *Tex Med* 2001; **97**: 50–8.

18 Larrieu S, Letenneur L, Orgogozo J *et al.* Incidence and outcome of mild cognitive impairment in a population-based prospective cohort. *Neurology* 2002; **59**: 1594–9.

19 Celsis P. Age-related cognitive decline, mild cognitive impairment or preclinical Alzheimer's disease? *Ann Med* 2000; **32**: 6–14.

20 Data on file. Pfizer.

21 Scottish Intercollegiate Guidelines Network (SIGN). Interventions in the Management of Behavioural and Psychological Aspects of Dementia. Edinburgh: SIGN, 1998. *www.sign.ac.uk*

22 Dooley M, Lamb HM. Donepezil: a review of its use in Alzheimer's disease. *Drugs Aging* 2000; **16**: 199–226.

23 Kirby L, Lehmann P, Majeed A. Dementia in people aged 65 years and older: a growing problem? *Population Trends* 1998; **92**: 23–8.

24 DeLaGarza VW. Pharmacologic treatment of Alzheimer's disease: an update. *Am Fam Physician* 2003; **68**: 1365–72.

25 Kivipelto M, Helkala EL, Hanninen T *et al.* Midlife vascular risk factors and late-life mild cognitive impairment: a population-based study. *Neurology* 2001; **56**: 1683–9.

26 DeKosky ST. Pathology and pathways of Alzheimer's disease with an update on new developments in treatment. *J Am Geriatr Soc* 2003; **51**: S314–20.

27 Doody RS. Clinical profile of donepezil in the treatment of Alzheimer's disease. *Gerontology* 1999; **45(Suppl 1)**: 23–32.

28 Shinotoh H, Namba H, Fukushi K *et al.* Progressive loss of cortical acetylcholinesterase activity in association with cognitive decline in Alzheimer's disease: a positron emission tomography study. *Ann Neurol* 2000; **48**: 194–200.

29 Cummings JL, Back C. The cholinergic hypothesis of neuropsychiatric symptoms in Alzheimer's disease. *Am J Geriatr Psychiatry* 1998; **6**: S64–78.

30 Imbimbo BP. Pharmacodynamic-tolerability relationships of cholinesterase inhibitors for Alzheimer's disease. *CNS Drugs* 2001; **15**: 375–90.

31 Stewart R. Risk factors for dementia. Alzheimer's Disease International website; factsheet 9: *http://www.alz.co.uk*

32 Lindsay J, Laurin D, Verreault R *et al.* Risk factors for Alzheimer's disease: a prospective analysis from the Canadian Study of Health and Aging. *Am J Epidemiol* 2002; **156**: 445–53.

33 Wisniewski KE, Wisniewski HM, Wen GY. Occurrence of neuropathological changes and dementia of Alzheimer's disease in Down's syndrome. *Ann Neurol* 1985; **17**: 278–82.

34 Lemere CA, Blusztajn JK, Yamaguchi H *et al.* Sequence of deposition of heterogeneous amyloid beta-peptides and APO E in Down syndrome: implications for initial events in amyloid plaque formation. *Neurobiol Dis* 1996; **3**: 16–32.

35 Roman GC, Rogers SJ. Donepezil: a clinical review of current and emerging indications. *Expert Opin Pharmacother* 2004; **5**: 161–80.

36 Devanand D, Sano M, Tang M *et al.* Depressed mood and the incidence of Alzheimer's disease in the elderly living in the community. *Arch Gen Psychiatry* 1996; **53**: 175–82.

37 Barberger-Gateau P, Letenneur L, Deschamps V *et al.* Fish, meat, and risk of dementia: cohort study. *BMJ* 2002; **325**: 932–3.

38 Morris M, Evans D, Bienias J *et al.* Dietary intake of antioxidant nutrients and the risk of incident Alzheimer disease in a biracial community study. *JAMA* 2002; **287**: 3230–7.

39 Morris M, Evans D, Bienias J *et al.* Consumption of fish and n-3 fatty acids and risk of incident Alzheimer disease. *Arch Neurol* 2003; **60**: 940–6.

40 Engelhart M, Geerlings M, Ruitenberg A *et al.* Dietary intake of antioxidants and risk of Alzheimer disease. *JAMA* 2002; **287**: 3223–9.

41 Doody RS. Current treatments for Alzheimer's disease: cholinesterase inhibitors. *J Clin Psychiatry* 2003; **64(Suppl 9)**: 11–17.

42 Reisberg B, Doody R, Stoffler A *et al.* Memantine in moderate-to-severe Alzheimer's disease. *N Engl J Med* 2003; **348**: 1333–41.

43 Ferris SH. Evaluation of memantine for the treatment of Alzheimer's disease. *Expert Opin Pharmacother* 2003; **4**: 2305–13.

44 Sano M, Ernesto C, Thomas RG *et al.* A controlled trial of selegiline, alpha-tocopherol, or both as treatment for Alzheimer's disease. The Alzheimer's Disease Cooperative Study. *N Engl J Med* 1997; **336**: 1216–22.

Acknowledgements

Figure 5 is adapted from Kirby, *et al.* 1998.[23]

PATIENT NOTES
Dr Steve Illiffe

Introduction

All organs of the body can fail and the brain is no exception. We know that kidneys can fail, and in this case the treatment is dialysis or transplantation, but in brain failure of the kind described in this book – Alzheimer's disease – there is no such radical cure. Treatments exist, and are important (not least to the patient themselves). However, they do not modify the underlying disease that causes the brain to fail but instead relieve some of its symptoms. This is the first important point that we should note about the treatment of Alzheimer's disease.

What is Alzheimer's disease and what causes it?

Early in the nineteenth century when psychiatry was emerging as a medical science the dementias were thought of as either types of psychosis (like schizophrenia) or related to what we now refer to as learning disability. Later in the century 'senile dementia' was recognised as a memory disorder with a number of different subtypes. Alzheimer's disease – named after the physician who identified it as a distinct form of dementia – is one of these subtypes and has a characteristic pattern of structural and biochemical changes in the brain.

The causes of Alzheimer's disease are unclear, and the mechanisms of brain failure are complex, but scientific knowledge about brain activity has expanded enormously over recent decades and has directly led to the introduction of some novel treatments. This expansion of knowledge is accelerating, and as a consequence we can expect new generations of therapies to appear, which may offer improved symptom relief for many more people with Alzheimer's disease. Together with a better understanding of the psychological techniques that assist people with Alzheimer's disease, this advance in medical treatments is changing the approach to this debilitating disease. This hope for emerging treatment is the second major point to emphasise.

What happens during the typical course of Alzheimer's disease?

Brain failure of the Alzheimer's type occurs because brain cells (neurones) communicate less. Effective communication between brain cells is dependent upon transmitter chemicals released by one cell, sensed by another, and then cleared from the space

Alzheimer's disease has a characteristic pattern of structural and biochemical changes in the brain.

between the cells. The clearance of this chemical 'message' is essential if new messages are to be sent. If the release of transmitter chemicals is reduced, as it is in Alzheimer's disease, there are two theoretical ways to improve cell-to-cell communication. One is to stimulate the release of more transmitter chemicals, and the other is to slow down their clearance. The current generation of drugs that are available to reduce the symptoms of early Alzheimer's disease work mainly by slowing the clearance of one of these transmitter chemicals, although one drug acts by preventing the build up of toxic chemicals between cells. We will return to an account of how medication can help, after considering what happens in Alzheimer's disease as it progresses.

The initial loss of transmitter chemicals is slight, and the changes in the way people think, feel and behave are similarly small. Some forgetfulness is expected as we get older, and also when we are tired, overburdened or depressed, so the early losses in memory can be attributed to ageing or the stresses of everyday life. The person with the earliest changes of Alzheimer's disease can often compensate for them, covering up a forgotten name or explaining away their failure to work out change at the supermarket checkout, or to remember which bus gets them home. They may also sense that they are not thinking clearly, often talk about being muddled, and perhaps feel apprehensive or despondent as they notice their loss of skills.

As the levels of the transmitter chemical decline further, decisions become harder to make, complex tasks become more difficult, interest in people and events diminishes, and new ideas become harder to understand. Further loss results in short-term memory loss and difficulties with ordinary, taken-for-granted and routine activities like dressing, shaving, making a cup of tea or preparing a meal. The individual may become irritable, prone to repetitive questioning or actions, and may also become 'clingy'. Getting lost is a common problem, and acting inappropriately (going out in the wrong clothing for the weather, for example) or in a disinhibited way also emerge as additional problems. Some people with Alzheimer's disease may exhibit paranoid ideas and accuse others of stealing their property, or see things that are not actually there.

Progression of the disease results in loss of speech, increasing frailty, incontinence and inability to eat without help.

Further progression of the disease results in loss of speech, increasing frailty, incontinence and inability to eat without help. The individual becomes bed-bound and needs nursing care day and night. This typical course can take up to 10 years from recognition of the significance of the early symptoms, though the majority of older people with Alzheimer's disease will die from other causes before reaching this last phase of the disease.

Risk factors for Alzheimer's disease

Although there are some families in which Alzheimer's disease appears to be inherited, most people who develop the disease do so in later life, and the risk of the disease increases with age. Alcohol in excess seems to increase the risk, whilst education reduces it, and these factors may offer clues as to how we can prevent the disorder, at least in some people. More important, however, are the ways in we can recognise Alzheimer's disease at an early stage, and thus reduce its impact on individuals and their families. This is the third important point about the medical response to this disease. Later on in this book we will look at what you or your loved one can expect from your family doctor when treating this debilitating and distressing disease.

Most people who develop the disease do so in later life, and the risk of the disease increases with age.

2. Drug review – Donepezil (Aricept®)

Dr Eleanor Bull
CSF Medical Communications Ltd

Summary

Donepezil is an <u>acetylcholinesterase inhibitor</u> indicated for the symptomatic relief of mild-to-moderately severe Alzheimer's disease. By selectively targeting the acetylcholinesterase <u>enzyme</u>, donepezil inhibits the hydrolysis of <u>acetylcholine</u>, thus increasing its availability in the <u>synaptic cleft</u> and enhancing <u>cholinergic</u> neurotransmission. In clinical terms, patients can expect a stabilisation of their <u>cognitive</u> abilities, behavioural abnormalities and daily functioning following donepezil treatment. By stabilising symptoms, donepezil may also relieve the burden placed on the carers of patients with Alzheimer's disease. Donepezil has a prolonged <u>systemic half-life</u> and consequently, need only be administered once daily. This is in contrast to the other available drugs in this class and thus, may promote patient concordance. The limited drug–<u>drug interaction</u> profile of donepezil is of benefit when treating elderly patients, many of whom are likely to be taking concomitant medication for <u>comorbid</u> conditions. Donepezil is distinguishable from the alternative <u>cholinesterase inhibitors</u> by its good tolerability profile. The majority of side-effects are mild in severity and usually resolve with continued administration.

Introduction

To date, current pharmacological treatments for Alzheimer's disease do not tend to modify disease progression. Current symptomatic treatments, of which the cholinesterase inhibitors are by far the most effective, seek to compensate for the loss of cholinergic <u>neurones</u> in key brain areas by increasing cholinergic activity.

The cholinesterase inhibitors (e.g. tacrine,[a] donepezil, galantamine, rivastigmine) prevent the hydrolysis of acetylcholine in the <u>synapse</u> by inhibiting the acetylcholinesterase enzyme. This increases the availability

---

[a]Tacrine is not currently licensed in the UK.

The <u>cholinesterase inhibitors</u> prevent the hydrolysis of acetylcholine in the <u>synapse</u> by inhibiting the <u>acetylcholinesterase enzyme</u>.

of acetylcholine to postsynaptic receptors and thus potentiates cholinergic neurotransmission.[1] Consequently, these drugs may slow the rate of cognitive decline, normalise behaviour and exert a positive effect on mood and activities of daily living in patients with Alzheimer's disease. The most common side-effects associated with cholinesterase inhibitors are due to peripheral and central cholinergic over-stimulation and may include nausea, vomiting, diarrhoea, fatigue, muscle cramps and dizziness.[1]

Tacrine[b] was the first pharmacological agent to be approved for the treatment of Alzheimer's disease.[2] However, its use has been limited by reports of hepatotoxicity, gastrointestinal disturbance and the necessity for frequent laboratory monitoring and multiple daily dosing.[3] Rivastigmine – a pseudo-reversible inhibitor of acetylcholinesterase and butyrylcholinesterase – and galantamine – an acetylcholinesterase inhibitor with agonistic properties at the nicotinic receptor – must be administered twice daily, which may hinder patient concordance.

Donepezil is a reversible acetylcholinesterase inhibitor rationally designed for the symptomatic treatment of Alzheimer's disease following the discovery of the antidementive effects of tacrine. First introduced in 1997, donepezil is indicated for the treatment of mild-to-moderately severe Alzheimer's disease and has the advantage of once-daily administration. This article reviews the properties of donepezil and its efficacy in controlled clinical trials in the context of other available treatments for Alzheimer's disease.

Pharmacology

☞ *The chemistry of donepezil is of essentially academic interest and most healthcare professionals will, like you, skip this section.*

Chemistry

The chemical structure of donepezil hydrochloride is illustrated in Figure 1.[4] A piperidine-based acetylcholinesterase inhibitor, donepezil is chemically unrelated to the other acetylcholinesterase inhibitors.[3] Structure–activity studies have indicated that both the benzoyl-containing functional group and the N-benzylpiperidine moiety are the key features essential for the binding and inhibition of acetylcholinesterase.[5]

Figure 1. The chemical structure of donepezil hydrochloride ($C_{24}H_{29}NO_3HCl$).

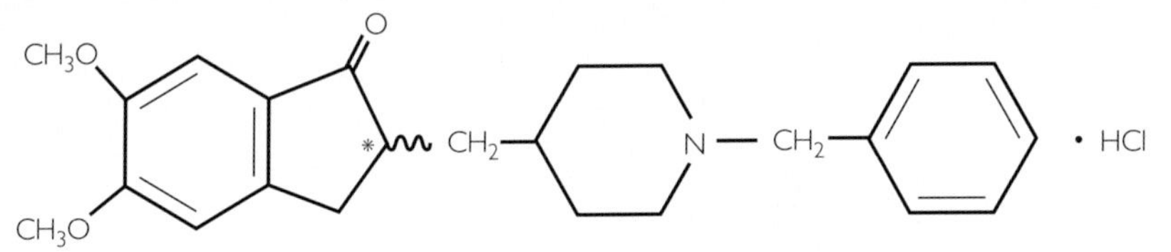

---

[b]Tacrine is not currently licensed in the UK.

Mechanism of action

Donepezil is a reversible, non-competitive inhibitor of acetylcholinesterase. By increasing the availability of intrasynaptic acetylcholine, donepezil enhances cholinergic function in the surviving neurones of patients with Alzheimer's disease.[6] Donepezil has a predominantly central mechanism of action and exerts maximal effects in the cortex and hippocampus of the brain.[7]

In vitro activity

Donepezil is more selective for acetylcholinesterase than butyrylcholinesterase in the central nervous system, based on its molecular structure and anionic interactions with the enzyme.[8] *In vitro* studies have shown that the potency and specificity of donepezil for acetylcholinesterase over butyrylcholinesterase is 1265:1.[8] Table 1 illustrates the potency of donepezil for acetylcholinesterase and butyrylcholinesterase, in terms of IC_{50}[c] values, compared with tacrine and heptylphysostigmine, a derivative of the early acetylcholinesterase inhibitor, physostigmine.[9]

☞ These preclinical data sections describe the results of the earliest phases of a drug's development (see Reader's Guide).

The relationship between the plasma concentration of donepezil and the extent of acetylcholinesterase inhibition is linear.[10] In mice, brain levels of acetylcholine were increased in a dose-dependent manner following donepezil administration, reaching approximately 50% at the highest dosage tested (32 mg/kg).[9] Similarly, in humans the plasma concentration of donepezil is dose-related and plateaus at 50 ng/mL, which corresponds to 80–90% acetylcholinesterase inhibition.[11] A clinical effect is observed when acetylcholinesterase inhibition exceeds 60%.[6]

Experiments conducted in both young and aged rats examined the effect of donepezil, at doses of 1.25–5 mg/kg, on acetylcholinesterase activity in various tissues.[12] In young rats, the inhibition of acetylcholinesterase activity was dose dependent and was less pronounced in the heart and small intestine. The inhibition of acetylcholinesterase activity elicited by donepezil in the brain, erythrocytes and pectoral muscle of aged rats was more potent than that in young animals. This suggests that the differential effect of donepezil

Table 1. *In vitro* inhibition (IC_{50}) of the enzymes involved in acetylcholine inhibition.[9]

Enzyme	Donepezil	Icopezil	Tacrine	Heptylphysostigmine
Acetylcholinesterase (nM)	19 ± 7	0.33 ± 0.09	108 ± 7	110 ± 20
Butyrylcholinesterase (nM)	4100 ± 1800	7200 ± 1200	29 ± 2	17

NB. Icopezil is a benzylpiperidine compound, currently unlicensed.

[c]IC_{50} – concentration in nM required to inhibit the activity of the enzyme by 50%.

between young and aged animals is attributable to differences in tissue concentrations of donepezil.

In vivo *activity*

Testament to its central selectivity, when administered to rats at high concentrations, donepezil demonstrates a greater potency to induce tremors, a central effect, than peripherally mediated salivation.[9]

Donepezil has been shown to improve cognitive performance in a number of animal models of cholinergic deficiency. In hypocholinergic rats resulting from lesions of the nucleus basalis magnocellularis (NBM), donepezil alleviated the lesion-induced deficits in the passive avoidance response at doses greater than 0.125 mg/kg.[13] In contrast, tacrine had no effect on these deficits. Similarly, donepezil (0.5 mg/kg) reversed the impairment of acquisition in the water maze paradigm – a test of working memory – induced by lesions of the medial septum, whilst tacrine had no effect.[13] Furthermore, ovariectomised rats demonstrated enhanced performance in visual recognition and spatial memory tasks 1 week following initiation of donepezil treatment.[14]

Human studies

Effects on brain function

The effect of donepezil on functional brain activity was examined in a blinded placebo-controlled pilot study in 28 patients with mild-to-moderate Alzheimer's disease.[15] Patients received donepezil, 10 mg daily, or placebo, for a period of 24 weeks, after which time, regional brain glucose metabolism – a marker of functional brain activity – was assessed by positron emission tomography (PET) with radiolabelled [2-^{18}F] fluoro- 2-deoxyglucose. At week 24, mean brain glucose metabolism in striatal axial slices was maintained within 0.5% of baseline activity with donepezil but deteriorated by 10.4% in placebo-treated patients (p=0.015; Figure 2). Baseline changes in regional cerebral glucose metabolism at this time point also favoured donepezil in four predefined regions of interest; the right parietal lobe (p=0.044), the left temporal lobe (p=0.045) and the left and right frontal lobes (p=0.026 and p=0.018, respectively).

In a magnetic resonance imaging (MRI) study in 67 patients with mild-to-moderate Alzheimer's disease, the effect of donepezil on neuronal markers and hippocampal volume was compared with that of placebo.[16] Donepezil – 5 mg daily titrated up to 10 mg after 28 days – or placebo, were administered for a period of 24 weeks. Donepezil-treated patients showed significantly smaller mean decreases in total and right hippocampal volumes compared with the placebo group. In conjunction with this, mean Alzheimer's Disease Assessment Scale - cognitive subscale (ADAS-cog) scores were significantly improved following donepezil at weeks 6, 12, 18 and 24 compared with placebo (p<0.05).

> Donepezil-treated patients showed significantly smaller mean decreases in total and right hippocampal volumes compared with the placebo group.

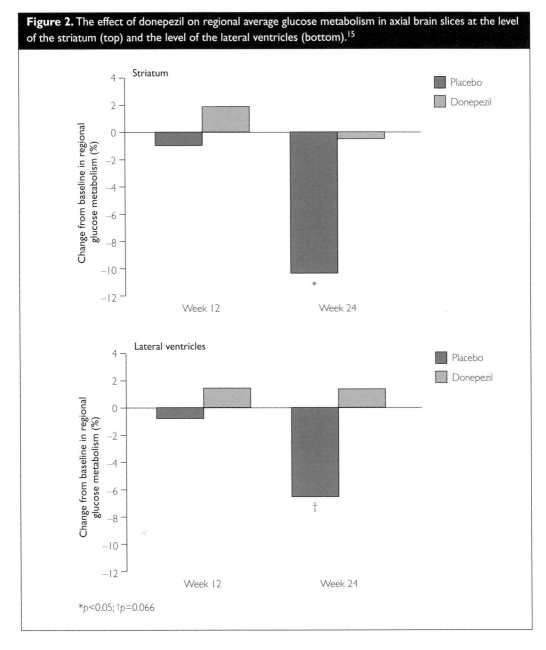

Figure 2. The effect of donepezil on regional average glucose metabolism in axial brain slices at the level of the striatum (top) and the level of the lateral ventricles (bottom).[15]

*p<0.05; †p=0.066

The latency of the P300 component of cognitive event-related potentials is altered following cholinergic dysfunction. On this basis, a study in 60 patients with mild-to-moderate Alzheimer's disease investigated the effect of donepezil, rivastigmine or vitamin E on P300 latency, measured using scalp electrodes.[17] After a 26-week treatment period, P300 latencies were increased by 7.4 msec in those patients receiving vitamin E, 2000 IU daily, an effect which was positively correlated with the worsening of neuropsychological scores. In contrast, patients receiving donepezil, 5–10 mg daily, and rivastigmine, 1.5–12 mg daily, showed significant reductions in P300 latencies (15.3 and 22.0 msec for donepezil and rivastigmine, respectively). These improvements in latencies were associated with higher Wechsler Adult Intelligence scores and lower ADAS-cog scores (r=0.72).

Pharmacokinetics

The pharmacokinetics of a drug are of interest to healthcare professionals because it is important for them to understand the action of a drug on the body over a period of time.

The pharmacokinetic properties of donepezil are presented in Table 2. Donepezil is well absorbed following oral administration and, as reflected by its t_{max} value, shows a slower rate of absorption than the other cholinesterase inhibitors (0.8–1.7 and 0.5–1.5 hours for rivastigmine and galantamine, respectively).[8] The more gradual onset of pharmacodynamic activity of donepezil is consistent with its lower potential to cause cholinergic side-effects.[18] This is in contrast to rivastigmine, which has a shorter t_{max} and therefore an increased propensity to elicit cholinergic side-effects.[18] The pharmacokinetics of donepezil are dose-proportional following single and multiple doses to healthy volunteers with no evidence of a time of dosing effect.[10,19,20] Food does not affect the absorption characteristics of donepezil, unlike rivastigmine and galantamine, which show decreased absorption when administered with food.[8]

The prolonged systemic half-life of donepezil of 48–78 hours is sufficient to permit once-daily dosing. This is in contrast to rivastigmine and galantamine which do not remain in the body as long and must be administered twice daily.[10,21] In the elderly, the elimination half-life of donepezil is approximately twice that in young adults (103.8 and 59.7 hours, respectively), although no dosage adjustment is necessary in these patients.[3] The predominant route of elimination of donepezil is

Table 2. The pharmacokinetic properties of donepezil at a dosage of 5–10 mg.[6,18]	
Pharmacokinetic parameter	
Absolute oral bioavailability (%)	90–100
t_{max} (hours)	3–4
C_{max} (mg/L)	7.2–25.6
Plasma protein binding (%)	96
$t_{1/2}$ (hours)	47.9–78.4
Plasma clearance (L/hour)	7–10
Volume of distribution (L)	800–900
AUC (µg.L/hour)	500–1000

AUC, area under the concentration-time curve; t_{max}, time to reach maximum drug plasma concentration (C_{max}); $t_{1/2}$, elimination half life.

renal, with 79% of a single 5 mg oral dose excreted in the urine and 21% in the faeces.[22] In patients with compromised hepatic or renal function, the pharmacokinetics of donepezil are unaltered with no need for dosage adjustment in this population.[23,24]

Donepezil is metabolised by the cytochrome P450 (CYP) enzymes, CYP2D6 and CYP3A4, and undergoes extensive first-pass metabolism.[8] As a result, donepezil may interact with those drugs metabolised by both CYP enzymes and those drugs which affect the cholinergic system, although no clinically significant interactions have been reported with digoxin, theophylline, warfarin, ketoconazole or cimetidine.[3] Drugs which induce CYP2D6 and CYP3A4 enzymes (e.g. phenytoin, carbamazepine, dexamethasone, rifampicin and phenobarbital) may increase the rate of elimination of donepezil.[4]

Clinical efficacy

Dose-ranging studies

A 12-week dose-ranging study by the Donepezil Study Group was conducted in 161 patients with mild-to-moderate Alzheimer's disease with a Mini-Mental State Examination (MMSE) score of between 10 and 26 and a Clinical Dementia Rating (CDR) of 1 or 2.[25] In addition to assessing the cognitive effects of daily administrations of donepezil, 1, 3 or 5 mg, compared with placebo, the study also examined the relationship between plasma donepezil concentration, red blood cell acetylcholinesterase activity and clinical response. After 12 weeks, ADAS-cog scores were significantly improved in those patients receiving donepezil, 5 mg, compared with placebo-treated patients ($p \leq 0.05$; Figure 3). This trend was echoed by the clinical decline values, which showed a 50% improvement following the highest dosage of donepezil (11 vs 20% for 5 mg and placebo groups, respectively). Furthermore, there was a significant correlation between the plasma concentration of donepezil and the degree of acetylcholinesterase inhibition, with a plateau of inhibition (76–84%) reached at plasma concentrations above 50 ng/mL. The plasma concentration of donepezil was also positively correlated with ADAS-cog ($p=0.014$), MMSE ($p=0.023$) and patient-assessed quality of life scores ($p=0.037$). The adverse event profile was similar at all three dosages tested and was comparable to that reported following placebo administration.

In an extension of this trial, 133 patients from the original study were recruited into an open-label study of up to 254 weeks duration.[26] For the first 6–9 months of the study, ADAS-cog and Clinical Dementia Rating-Sum of the Boxes (CDR-SB) scores continued to improve, although scores gradually deteriorated beyond this time point. Adverse events were mild and transient and resolved with no need for dosage adjustment.

☛ *Dose-ranging studies are particularly important to ensure that the optimum dose of a drug can be determined in order that benefit can be realised with the least risk of side-effects.*

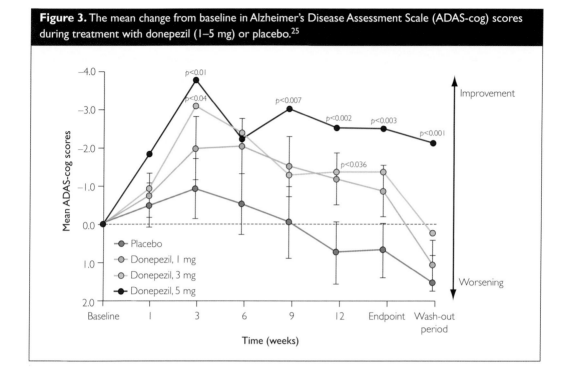

Figure 3. The mean change from baseline in Alzheimer's Disease Assessment Scale (ADAS-cog) scores during treatment with donepezil (1–5 mg) or placebo.[25]

Placebo-controlled trials

The effectiveness of donepezil has been assessed in a number of placebo-controlled clinical trials, summarised in Table 3.[27–35] ADAS-cog scores have commonly been used to assess the effect of drug treatment on the cognitive impairment associated with Alzheimer's disease. Changes in ADAS-cog scores should be weighted against the usual annual decline in ADAS-cog of 7–9 points in these patients.

An open-label extension of two placebo-controlled trials[27,28] further examined the effect of donepezil up to 144 weeks following treatment initiation.[36] During the original studies, all patients (n=763) had received donepezil at a daily dosage of 5 mg which was increased to 10 mg after 6 weeks. Following a 3-week placebo wash-out period, donepezil-related benefits were sustained above baseline values for an additional 24 weeks of open-label treatment. Furthermore, ADAS-cog score improvements were evident following 10 mg donepezil for up to 108 weeks of open-label treatment. At this dose, mean ADAS-cog scores remained at, or improved from, baseline for almost a year of treatment (mean change from baseline score at week 51, +0.57 *vs* +1.92 and +1.93 for placebo and 5 mg donepezil, respectively).

A long-term double-blind study examined the effects of donepezil (5 mg daily for 28 days, increased to 10 mg thereafter) or placebo in 286 patients with possible or probable Alzheimer's disease for a 1-year period.[33] The percentage of patients completing the trial was similar for donepezil and placebo (66.9 and 67.4%, respectively). The effectiveness

ADAS-cog score improvements were evident following 10 mg donepezil for up to 108 weeks of open-label treatment.

Table 3. Summary of placebo-controlled trials examining donepezil for the treatment of mild-to-moderate Alzheimer's disease.[27–35]

Study	Design	Disease severity	Donepezil dose	Outcomes
Rogers et al., 1998[27]	Double-blind Multicentre 12 weeks 3-week wash-out n=468	Mild-to-moderate	5 or 10 mg/day	• ADAS-cog score improved following donepezil, 5 and 10 mg (2.5 and 3.1 units, respectively; $p<0.001$ vs placebo). • CIBIC plus score improved following donepezil, 5 and 10 mg (32 and 38%, respectively; $p≤0.008$ vs placebo [18%]). • MMSE score improved following donepezil, 5 and 10 mg (1.0 and 1.3 units, respectively; $p≤0.004$ vs placebo). • Adverse event profile of donepezil comparable with that of placebo.
Rogers et al., 1998[28]	Double-blind Multicentre 24 weeks 6-week wash-out n=473	Mild-to-moderate	5 or 10 mg/day	• ADAS-cog score improved following both doses of donepezil at weeks 12, 18 and 24 ($p≤0.001$ vs placebo). • Clinician global rating improved following both doses of donepezil ($p≤0.005$ at endpoint vs placebo). • MMSE and CDR-SB scores superior following both doses of donepezil ($p≤0.0007$ vs placebo). • No consistent effect on patient-rated quality of life. • Cholinergic side-effects more frequent following 10 mg donepezil ($p≤0.05$ vs 5 mg and placebo).
Burns et al., 1999[29]	Double-blind Multicentre 24 weeks 6-week wash-out n=818	Mild-to-moderate	5 or 10 mg/day	• ADAS-cog score improved following both doses of donepezil ($p≤0.002$ vs placebo at endpoint). • CIBIC plus score improved following both doses of donepezil ($p≤0.008$ vs placebo at endpoint). • CDR-SB score improved following both doses of donepezil ($p≤0.035$ vs placebo at endpoint). • Well tolerated across all treatment groups.

ADAS-cog, Alzheimer's Disease Assessment Scale; ADFACS, Alzheimer's Disease Functional Assessment and Change Scale; BADLS, Bristol Activities of Daily Living Scale; CDR-SB, Clinical Dementia Rating-Sum of the Boxes; CGIC, Clinical Global Impression of Change; CIBIC plus, Clinician's Interview-Based Impression of Change including caregiver information; GBS, Gottfries-Bråne-Steen scale; MMSE, Mini-Mental State Examination; NPI-NH, Neuropsychiatric Inventory–Nursing Home version.

Table 3. Continued

Study	Design	Disease severity	Donepezil dose	Outcomes
Rogers *et al.*, Gauthier *et al.*, 2002[30]	Double-blind Double-blind Multicentre 24 weeks n=207	Mild-to-Moderate	5 or 5 mg/day for first 28 days and 10 mg/day thereafter	• ADAS-cog score improved following • MMSE scores improved following donepezil (*p*<0.0002 *vs* placebo). • Disability assessment for dementia deteriorated following placebo *vs* donepezil (mean difference –9.25; *p*<0.0001). • NPI score superior to placebo at weeks 4 and 24 (*p*=0.0022). • Similar adverse event profile.
Homma *et al.*, 2000[31]	Double-blind Multicentre 24 weeks n=268	Mild-to-moderate	5 mg/day	• CGIC (Japanese variant) score improved following donepezil (52 *vs* 22% following placebo; *p*=0.000). • Similar adverse event profiles in donepezil and placebo groups – mild, mostly gastrointestinal.
Tariot *et al.*, 2001[32]	Double-blind Multicentre Nursing-home setting 24 weeks n=208	Mean MMSE score 14.4	5 mg/day for first 28 days and 10 mg/day thereafter	• NPI-NH scores not significantly different between donepezil and placebo groups. • CDR-SB score improved following donepezil at week 24 (*p*<0.05 *vs* placebo). • MMSE scores improved following donepezil at weeks 8, 16, 20 (*p*<0.05 *vs* placebo for each timepoint). • Adverse event profiles similar between treatment groups. • 11% of donepezil and 18% of placebo group withdrew due to adverse events.
Winblad *et al.*, 2001[33]	Double-blind Multinational 1 year n=286	Mild-to-moderate	5 mg/day for first 28 days and 10 mg/day thereafter	• Change in GBS score from baseline to week 52, 7.3 *vs* 13.5 for donepezil and placebo, respectively (*p*=0.014). • MMSE score improved following donepezil at study endpoint (*p*<0.001 *vs* placebo). • Adverse event profiles similar between treatment groups.

ADAS-cog, Alzheimer's Disease Assessment Scale; ADFACS, Alzheimer's Disease Functional Assessment and Change Scale; BADLS, Bristol Activities of Daily Living Scale; CDR-SB, Clinical Dementia Rating-Sum of the Boxes; CGIC, Clinical Global Impression of Change; CIBIC plus, Clinician's Interview-Based Impression of Change including caregiver information; GBS, Gottfries-Bråne-Steen scale; MMSE, Mini-Mental State Examination; NPI-NH, Neuropsychiatric Inventory–Nursing Home version.

Table 3. Continued

Study	Design	Disease severity	Donepezil dose	Outcomes
Mohs et al., 2001[34]	Double-blind Multicentre 1 year n=431	Mild-to-moderate	5 mg/day for first 28 days and 10 mg/day thereafter	• Time to clinically evident functional decline (Kaplan–Meier) extended following donepezil (survival curves different; $p=0.002$ vs placebo, log-rank test). • MMSE scores higher at endpoint following donepezil ($p<0.001$ vs placebo). • ADFACS scores improved from baseline following donepezil (Figure 4).
Courtney et al., 2004[35]	Double-blind Multicentre 12-week run-in followed by indefinite treatment duration n=565	Mild-to-moderate	5 mg/day for first 12 weeks and 5 or 10 mg/day thereafter	• Mean MMSE scores improved significantly following donepezil treatment over the first 2 years (0.8 points better than placebo; $p<0.001$). • Mean BADLS scores improved significantly following donepezil over the first 2 years (1.0 points better than placebo; $p<0.0001$). • No change in institutionalisation rate following 3 years of treatment with donepezil (42 vs 44%; $p=0.4$ vs placebo). • No change in progression of disability after 3 years of treatment with donepezil (58 vs 59%; $p=0.04$ vs placebo).

ADAS-cog, Alzheimer's Disease Assessment Scale; ADFACS, Alzheimer's Disease Functional Assessment and Change Scale; BADLS, Bristol Activities of Daily Living Scale; CDR-SB, Clinical Dementia Rating-Sum of the Boxes; CGIC, Clinical Global Impression of Change; CIBIC plus, Clinician's Interview-Based Impression of Change including caregiver information; GBS, Gottfries-Bråne-Steen scale; MMSE, Mini-Mental State Examination; NPI-NH, Neuropsychiatric Inventory–Nursing Home version.

of treatment, assessed using the Gottfries-Bråne-Steen (GBS) scale – a global assessment for dementia – was greater following donepezil at weeks 24, 36 and 52 ($p<0.05$ for all time points vs placebo). The least-squares mean change from baseline in the GBS intellectual impairment score was 3.6 following donepezil compared with 7.3 following placebo ($p=0.004$ at week 52). MMSE and Activities of Daily Living (ADL) scores were similarly affected at these time points, favouring donepezil over placebo ($p<0.02$). The adverse event profile was similar for donepezil and placebo and side-effects were commonly mild and transient in nature.

The long-term functional effects of donepezil treatment (5 mg daily for 28 days, increased to 10 mg thereafter) in 431 patients with mild-to-moderate Alzheimer's disease were examined in a year-long study.[34] The mean change from baseline to study endpoint in the Alzheimer's Disease Functional Assessment and Change Scale (ADFACS) favoured donepezil over placebo for both instrumental and basic ADL ($p=0.001$ and $p<0.001$ respectively [Figure 4]).

The Aricept Wash-out and Rechallenge (AWARE) study examined the effect of donepezil rechallenge in 202 patients with mild-to-moderate Alzheimer's disease who were initially unresponsive to donepezil treatment.[37] Those patients achieving 'no apparent clinical benefit' following a 12–24-week open-label donepezil treatment period were selected for a double-blind extension and received donepezil, 10 mg per day, or placebo for a further 24 weeks. Those patients continuing with donepezil showed significantly different MMSE and Neuropsychiatry Inventory (NPI) scale scores compared with placebo (treatment differences of –1.13 and 3.16 for MMSE and NPI scores, respectively; $p<0.05$).[37] This study illustrates the potential benefits of persisting with a donepezil treatment regimen, even when the initial response to treatment appears disappointing.

The longest placebo-controlled trial conducted to date, the AD2000 study, examined the efficacy of donepezil in 565 patients with mild-to-moderate Alzheimer's disease, with double-blind treatment continuing for as long as it was deemed appropriate.[35] Patients enrolled into this study underwent a 12-week run-in period during which time they received once-daily treatment with either donepezil, 5 mg, or placebo, before undergoing a second randomisation to either long-term treatment with donepezil, 5 or 10 mg/day, or placebo. After 60 weeks of treatment,

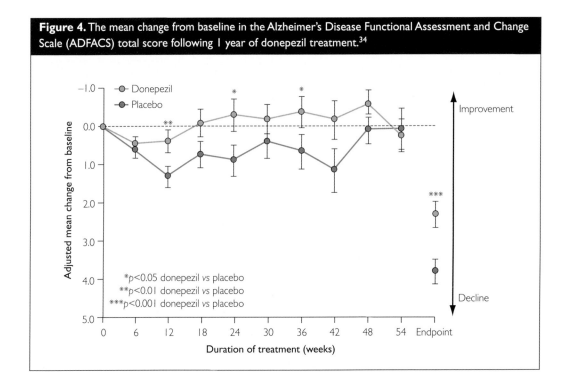

Figure 4. The mean change from baseline in the Alzheimer's Disease Functional Assessment and Change Scale (ADFACS) total score following 1 year of donepezil treatment.[34]

*$p<0.05$ donepezil vs placebo
**$p<0.01$ donepezil vs placebo
***$p<0.001$ donepezil vs placebo

the offer of indefinite treatment was extended, if approved by the physician, caregiver and the patient themselves. Patients also underwent a 4-week drug-free wash-out period after every 48 weeks of active treatment. Significantly fewer donepezil- than placebo-treated patients completed the 12-week run-in phase (89 *vs* 95%; *p*=0.007). This difference was attributed to the higher incidence of adverse events associated with donepezil treatment (6 *vs* 1%; *p*=0.001). However, from week 13 onwards, the number of premature discontinuations from the study was comparable between treatment groups, with 83% of donepezil- and 82% of placebo-treated patients remaining on their allocated treatment at 60 weeks. The rate of institutionalisation and the progression of disability were not affected by donepezil over a 3-year period of treatment (42 *vs* 44% and 58 *vs* 59%, for donepezil and placebo, respectively; *p*=0.4 for both comparisons). Over the 12-week run-in period, MMSE scores improved from baseline by an average of 0.9 points following donepezil treatment, compared with no change following placebo (*p*-value not reported). However, over 2 years, the MMSE score of donepezil-treated group averaged 0.8 points higher than placebo-treated patients (*p*<0.0001). Similarly, functional ability as determined by the Bristol Activities of Daily Living Scale (BADLS) averaged 1.0 points higher in the donepezil group (*p*<0.0001 *vs* placebo). The total number of serious adverse events and deaths were similar between treatment groups (10 *vs* 8% and 22 *vs* 18% for donepezil and placebo, respectively; *p*=0.4 and *p*=0.2).

The study also included an economic evaluation of costs incurred by the NHS, social services and privately.[35] The mean annual cost per patient resident in the community for 11 formal health and social services was £498 higher following donepezil treatment compared with placebo treatment (*p*=0.16). Since this analysis did not include the cost of drug acquisition or institutionalisation, the largest extra cost was attributed to overnight hospital stays (£825 *vs* £439 per year; *p*=0.09). Overall, active caregiver daily time input was 0.2 hours less (*p*=0.2) and passive care time 0.4 hours less (*p*=0.4) in those patients treated with donepezil. Thus, the AD2000 study did not find any evidence that the costs of caring for patients with Alzheimer's dementia in the community are reduced by donepezil.

> The rate of institutionalisation and the progression of disability were not affected by donepezil over a 3-year period of treatment.

Meta-analysis

A meta-analysis of ten randomised, placebo-controlled trials of donepezil (two of which are currently unpublished) included a total of 2376 patients with mild-to-moderate Alzheimer's disease.[38] All studies were of 12 or 24 weeks' duration and patients received either placebo or donepezil, 5 or 10 mg/day. All studies, with the exception of one, used ADAS-cog scores as the primary efficacy evaluation. Overall, patients who received donepezil, 5 or 10 mg/day, demonstrated significantly better ADAS-cog scores at all time points compared with placebo-treated patients (*p*<0.001 [Figure 5]). The magnitude of the response was consistently greater in those patients treated with 10 mg daily doses of

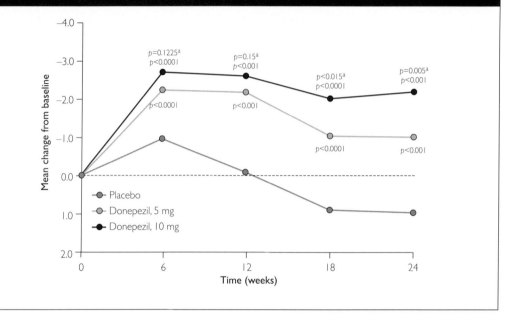

Figure 5. Mean change from baseline in Alzheimer's Disease Assessment Scale-cognitive subscale (ADAS-cog) score for patients with mild-to-moderate Alzheimer's disease treated with donepezil, 5 and 10 mg/day, and placebo. Data taken from a fixed-effects, meta-analysis of ten placebo-controlled studies.[38] [a]*p*-value for donepezil, 10 mg/day, *vs* donepezil, 5 mg/day.

The odds of showing an improvement in CIBIC-plus scores were approximately twice as great with donepezil than with placebo.

donepezil than those receiving the 5 mg daily dose, and this difference reached <u>statistical significance</u> by week 18 and was maintained to week 24 (*p*=0.015 and *p*=0.005, respectively). The odds of showing an improvement in Clinician's Interview-Based Impression of Change (CIBIC-plus) scores were approximately twice as great with donepezil, 5 or 10 mg/day, than with <u>placebo</u> and reached significance at all time points evaluated (odds ratios at week 24: 1.89 and 2.05 for donepezil, 5 and 10 mg/day, respectively; *p*<0.001 *vs* placebo). Study completion rates did not differ significantly between treatment groups (83.8, 76.1 and 83.9% for donepezil, 5 and 10 mg/day, and placebo, respectively), with <u>adverse events</u> the most common reason reported for treatment discontinuation (6.3, 13.9 and 5.8%, respectively; *<u>p</u>*-value not reported). Nausea, diarrhoea, headache, insomnia and vomiting occurred most frequently amongst those patients receiving the 10 mg daily dose of donepezil (*p*<0.01 *vs* placebo and donepezil, 5 mg/day).

Comparative clinical trials

Donepezil *vs* galantamine

The clinical <u>efficacy</u> of donepezil was compared with that of galantamine in a multinational study of 12 weeks' duration in 120 patients with mild-to-moderate disease.[39] Donepezil was administered at a dosage of up to 10 mg once daily and galantamine was given twice daily at 12 mg. Both physicians and caregivers reported greater overall satisfaction following donepezil at weeks 4, 12 and at <u>endpoint</u> (physicians score –26.8 *vs* 25.2 points at endpoint for donepezil and galantamine, respectively; *p*<0.001). In terms of <u>cognitive</u> improvement, measured using the <u>ADAS-cog</u> scale, donepezil was more effective than galantamine at week 12 (*p*≤0.01; Figure 6). ADL scores were similarly affected and showed greater improvement following donepezil treatment than with galantamine at weeks 4, 12 and at the study endpoint (*p*<0.05). Adverse events were mild-to-moderate for both treatment groups, but gastrointestinal symptoms occurred more frequently following galantamine (46%) than donepezil (25%).

In a comparative year-long study conducted by the Galantamine-GBR-2 Study Group, 182 patients with Alzheimer's disease and a MMSE score of 9–18, received either galantamine or donepezil. The dose of galantamine was escalated from 4 mg twice daily during weeks 1–4, to 8 mg twice daily for weeks 5–13. At 13 weeks, the dose could be increased to 12 mg twice daily at the investigator's discretion. Donepezil was administered as a daily dose of 5 mg, with the option to increase, if tolerated, to 10 mg after 4 weeks.[40] The BADLS highlighted no differences between the two treatments from <u>baseline</u> up to 52 weeks (mean change from baseline of 2.67 and 2.46 for donepezil and galantamine, respectively). Similarly, there was no treatment difference in terms of the change in MMSE total scores (mean change from baseline of 2.54 and 2.18 for donepezil and galantamine, respectively). The change in cognition in the total population, as measured by the

> Both physicians and caregivers reported greater overall satisfaction following donepezil, compared with galantamine, at weeks 4, 12 and endpoint.

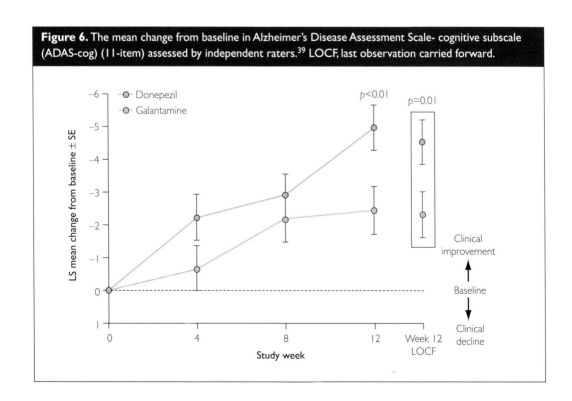

Figure 6. The mean change from baseline in Alzheimer's Disease Assessment Scale- cognitive subscale (ADAS-cog) (11-item) assessed by independent raters.[39] LOCF, last observation carried forward.

ADAS-cog scale, was again comparable between groups, with donepezil-treated patients exhibiting a decline of 3.43 compared with 2.22 in the galantamine group. Adverse events were similar between treatment groups and were mild-to-moderate in severity.

Donepezil *vs* rivastigmine

An open-label study in 111 patients with mild-to-moderate disease compared the efficacy of donepezil, up to 10 mg daily, with that of rivastigmine, up to 6 mg twice daily, over a 12-week period.[41] A greater number of donepezil-treated patients completed the study (89.3 *vs* 69.1% for donepezil and rivastigmine, respectively; *p*=0.009). Of those completing the study, 87.5% of patients receiving donepezil remained on the maximum approved dose at the last study visit, compared with 47.3% of rivastigmine patients. Furthermore, a higher proportion of rivastigmine-treated patients discontinued treatment due to intolerable side-effects (21.8 *vs* 10.7% for rivastigmine and donepezil, respectively). Donepezil was rated as superior to rivastigmine by physicians and caregivers in terms of satisfaction and ease of use (*p*<0.0001). Although both treatments elicited comparable improvements in ADAS-cog scores at weeks 4 and 12, donepezil treatment was associated with improved tolerability and a superior discontinuation rate.

Efficacy in clinical practice

The effectiveness and tolerability of donepezil in clinical practice is particularly pertinent considering the patient concordance issues associated with diseases of dementia.

An open-label study of 12 weeks' duration examined the effect of donepezil in a community-based sample of 1113 patients with mild-to-moderate Alzheimer's disease.[42] In common with many studies, the initial daily donepezil dosage of 5 mg was increased to 10 mg after 28 days at the physician's discretion. A large number of patients were receiving concomitant medications and 67% had a comorbid medical condition at study entry. A high proportion of patients completed the study (88.9%), with 5% withdrawing as a result of adverse events. Following donepezil treatment, cognitive function improved from baseline at weeks 4 and 12 (*p*<0.0001) and the mean change from the baseline MMSE score was +1.73 (*p*<0.0001). Patients also showed marked improvements in social interaction, engagement and interest, as assessed by the caregiver (20% improvement from baseline at week 1, increasing to 50% at week 12; *p*<0.0001).

> Following donepezil, patients showed marked improvements in social interaction, engagement and interest, as assessed by the caregiver.

A community-based, open-label study of similar size and duration was conducted in multiple centres across the US.[43] Patients (n=1035) with mild-to-moderate possible or probable Alzheimer's disease and a mean MMSE score of 19.8, had at least one comorbid medical condition or were taking concomitant medication. Following donepezil treatment, 5 mg daily increasing to 10 mg after 28 days, the mean MMSE score increased by 1.54 points from baseline (*p*<0.0001). The majority of adverse events were mild in severity and were unaffected by concomitant medication. Of particular note was the absence of a correlation between the incidence of gastrointestinal side-effects and the number of patients taking aspirin or other non-steroidal anti-inflammatory drugs concomitant with donepezil.

Post-marketing surveillance of donepezil, 5 or 10 mg once daily, conducted in 2092 patients with a mean MMSE score of 17.8, identified global improvements in clinical ratings after a 3-month period of administration.[44] Both MMSE and Nurses' Observational Scale for Geriatric patients (NOSGER) scores were significantly improved following donepezil (p=0.001 and p<0.001 for MMSE and NOSGER scores, respectively). Adverse events were reported in 12% of patients, with peripheral cholinergic effects the most frequent.

In the UK, an open-label study of donepezil was conducted in 80 patients with mild-to-moderate Alzheimer's disease in an elderly mental health clinic for a period of 18 months.[45] Patients received donepezil daily at 5 mg for the first 4 weeks, which was thereafter increased, if tolerated, to 10 mg. After 3 months of treatment, the mean improvement on the ADAS-cog scale was 1.07 from baseline (p=0.18), with 39% of patients improving by at least four points. MMSE scores at this time point were improved by an average of 0.96 points from baseline (p=0.02). With regard to neuropsychiatric symptoms, 37% of patients improved by four points or more on the NPI scale (p=0.001). The NPI improvements were sustained for up to 18 months and the ADAS-cog improvements for up to 6 months.

Most recently, the DONepezil in Alzheimer's Disease (DONALD) study examined the effect of donepezil, 5 or 10 mg/day, over 24 weeks in a group of out-patients with mild-to-moderate Alzheimer's disease.[46] Of the 237 patients who received donepezil treatment, 186 (79%) completed the study and the average duration of treatment was 169 days. Of the 21% who discontinued treatment prematurely, adverse events were the main reason cited, and accounted for 57% of all discontinuations. Following donepezil treatment, mean MMSE scores improved from baseline by 1.6 points at week 12 and by 1.1 points at week 24 (p-values not reported). At week 24, 68% of patients had improved or remained stable relative to their baseline values (35% improved by ≥3 points on MMSE scale and 10% improved by ≥6 points; p-values not reported). For more than 80% of patients, global tolerability was rated as very good or good, although 73% of patients experienced at least one treatment-emergent adverse event (including cardiovascular events, agitation, nausea or vomiting and muscle cramps), most of which were mild-to-moderate in severity. Electrocardiogram (ECG) recordings, available for 134 patients, detected no significant differences in heart rate and the mean PQ interval between donepezil and placebo treatment groups.

An analysis of data from the US, derived from the Minimum Data Set (MDS; n=174,659) – a standardised, clinically based, nursing-home resident assessment instrument – examined the use of donepezil for the treatment of Alzheimer's disease in clinical practice.[47] The overall incidence of donepezil use amongst patients with mild-to-moderate Alzheimer's dementia was 30% amongst newly admitted patients and 19% amongst long-stay residents. Of these patients, the proportion persisting with donepezil treatment after 6 months was 44.8% amongst newly admitted patients and 59.5% amongst long-stay residents. These relatively high withdrawal rates suggest that only a minority of nursing-home residents take donepezil chronically. The off-label use of donepezil for conditions other than Alzheimer's dementia was as high as 3% in this analysis.

Effect on delay to nursing home placement

Conducted in a community setting, the observational follow-up of three placebo-controlled trials and two open-label studies of donepezil examined the duration of treatment before nursing home placement became necessary for patients with Alzheimer's disease.[25–28,36] Data derived from interviews with caregivers and chart reviews of patients were available for 1115 patients.[48] Patients were grouped in terms of their donepezil use. Minimal use was defined as a dose of less than 5 mg/day for the required treatment period and maximal use was defined as a dose of at least 5 mg/day with greater than 80% compliance in both double-blind and open-label treatment periods. Donepezil was associated with significant delays in nursing home placement (44.7 months following minimal use and 66.1 months following maximal use of donepezil). Furthermore, there was a positive association between the length of treatment with donepezil and the delay in nursing home placement (r=0.604; *p*<0.001). If donepezil is taken at a daily dose of at least 5 mg for 9–12 months, the time gained before the first dementia-related nursing-home placement was estimated at 21.4 months, calculated as the difference between the times to first dementia-related nursing-home placement following minimal and maximal donepezil use. The delay in nursing-home placement following acetylcholinesterase therapy has been replicated in an open-label study in which the majority of patients were receiving long-term donepezil treatment.[49] During a 3-year follow-up period, 40% of untreated patients were admitted to a nursing home compared with 6% of treated patients.

> There was a positive association between the length of treatment with donepezil and the delay in nursing home placement.

Effect on caregiver burden

A nationwide survey conducted in the US, evaluated the scale of the care-giver burden in people caring for a total of 548 patients with Alzheimer's disease, receiving either donepezil or alternative treatments.[50] Donepezil was associated with significantly lower scores with regard to the overall difficulty of care giving (2.14 *vs* 2.37 for donepezil and non-donepezil-treated patients, respectively; *p*=0.004). These data included assisting with walking (*p*<0.001), emotional support (*p*<0.001) and managing behavioural problems (*p*=0.05). However, there was no difference in the time demands imposed on

> Donepezil was associated with significantly lower scores with regard to the overall difficulty of care giving.

carers as rated by the demand scale (3.35 *vs* 3.32 for donepezil and non-donepezil-treated patients).

The social and economic burden imposed on the caregiver is also reduced by donepezil therapy. A 1-year prospective northern European study of 286 patients with mild-to-moderate Alzheimer's disease evaluated the cost of treatment in terms of the impact on the caregiver.[51] Donepezil treatment reduced the caregiver burden by 400 hours over a 1-year period. The study estimated a total saving in treatment costs of US$1097 per patient following 1 year of donepezil intervention.

Special patient populations

Patients with comorbid cerebrovascular and Alzheimer's disease

The effect of donepezil in patients with concomitant cerebrovascular and Alzheimer's disease was examined in a German post-marketing surveillance study.[52] Of the 913 patients with mild-to-moderate Alzheimer's disease included in the study, 29.6% had documented cerebrovascular disease and 77.1% had previously received other antidementia drug therapies. Following 3 months of treatment with donepezil, 5 or 10 mg daily, MMSE scores had improved by an average of 2.2 points from baseline, this change measuring 2.4 points in patients with cerebrovascular disease and 2.1 points in patients without. Quality of life was improved in 70% of patients in total (72.5 and 69.6% of patients with and without cerebrovascular disease, respectively). Donepezil was generally well tolerated with adverse events affecting only 9.3% of the total population (11.2 and 7.9% in patients with and without cerebrovascular disease, respectively). These data suggest that donepezil has a similar efficacy and tolerability profile in Alzheimer's disease patients both with and without comorbid cerebrovascular disease.

Patients with Down syndrome

Down syndrome is a recognised risk factor for Alzheimer's disease. The effect of donepezil on symptoms of dementia in 30 patients with comorbid Alzheimer's disease and Down syndrome was examined in a 24-week placebo-controlled study.[53] In common with the majority of trials, the dosage of donepezil was initiated at 5 mg once daily and titrated to 10 mg after 4 weeks. Donepezil was well tolerated in this patient population, with no life-threatening side-effects reported. In terms of dementia rating, donepezil was associated with a non-significant reduction in the dementia scale commonly used to assess patients with learning disabilities, with 50% of donepezil-treated patients showing improvements compared with 31% of the placebo group. A follow-up study spanning 80 weeks, reviewed each patient in terms of their treatment options.[54] The rate of decline in dementia scores was less pronounced in those patients who were consistently treated with donepezil compared with those patients who had never received the drug (13.4 *vs* 25.6%, respectively, $p<0.001$).

Safety and tolerability

Donepezil treatment is generally associated with a low incidence of serious <u>adverse events</u>. <u>Cholinergic</u> side-effects, including nausea, vomiting, diarrhoea, anorexia, insomnia and muscle cramps have been widely reported, although tolerance to these effects usually develops with continued use (Table 4).[4,55]

This tolerability profile was confirmed in an integrated analysis of a number of phase 2/3 <u>placebo-controlled</u> trials encompassing a total of 1920 patients with mild-to-moderate Alzheimer's disease.[56] The majority of patients (94%) received donepezil at a dosage of 5 or 10 mg daily and 81% of patients were taking concomitant medication. The completion rate recorded in patients treated with donepezil was comparable with that in patients receiving <u>placebo</u> (79 *vs* 84% for donepezil and placebo, respectively). Overall, 11% of donepezil- and 7% of placebo-treated patients withdrew from the studies as a result of adverse events. In common with other studies, these adverse events included nausea, diarrhoea, headache, insomnia, dizziness, <u>rhinitis</u>, vomiting and fatigue. Donepezil was not associated with <u>hepatotoxicity</u> or abnormalities in any

Table 4. Adverse events reported in controlled clinical trials in at least 2% of patients receiving donepezil.[4]

Adverse event	Incidence of adverse events (%)	
	Placebo (n=355)	Donepezil (n=747)
Percentage of patients with any adverse event	72	74
Headache	9	10
Pain (various locations)	8	9
Accident	6	7
Fatigue	3	5
Syncope	1	2
Nausea	6	11
Diarrhoea	5	10
Vomiting	3	5
Anorexia	2	4
Ecchymosis	3	4
Weight loss	1	3
Muscle cramps	2	6
Arthritis	1	2
Insomnia	6	9
Dizziness	6	8
Depression	<1	3
Abnormal dreams	0	3
Somnolence	<1	2
Frequent urination	1	2

of the haematological, electrolytic or enzymatic laboratory tests performed.

A post-marketing pharmacovigilance study conducted in the UK followed 1762 patients receiving donepezil for Alzheimer's disease for a minimum of 6 months.[57] Consistent with other studies, the most common adverse events reported were nausea, diarrhoea, malaise, dizziness and insomnia. The study also highlighted a possible association between donepezil and increased agitation and aggression, which remains to be confirmed. No cardiac rhythm disturbances or liver disorders were reported.

As with all acetylcholinesterase inhibitors, following any interruption to donepezil therapy treatment should be restarted at the lowest dose and titrated accordingly, owing to the renewed susceptibility to side-effects.[58]

Pharmacoeconomics

Pharmacoeconomic analyses of the drugs used to treat Alzheimer's disease have reported difficulties in making inter-treatment comparisons as a result of different sources of data and outcome parameters.[59,60] Although direct comparisons of the different acetylcholinesterase inhibitors are lacking, the effect of donepezil compared with no pharmacological intervention has been evaluated. A 5-year costing of donepezil treatment in the UK, as evaluated by a modelling study in the context of a series of 6-month cycles, included both direct costs and the cost of informal care in patients with mild Alzheimer's disease.[61] In 1997, the total cost of caring for an Alzheimer's patient for the duration of the 5-year study period was £45,694 for donepezil and £44,278 for placebo, a difference of £1,416. The number of years expected before severe disease development was estimated at 1.69 following donepezil and 1.57 in patients having received no donepezil, an increase of 0.12 years.

There is evidence to suggest that donepezil reduces nursing home costs by delaying the time before nursing home placement becomes necessary.[62] This lower rate of nursing home placement may lead to a halving of associated costs compared with untreated patients ($p<0.01$).[63] The benefits of a once-daily dosage regimen may also impact on the overall cost of treatment with donepezil. By increasing patients' concordance with the dosage regimen, the clinical response to drug intervention may improve, which may ultimately reduce the overall costs of nursing home placement.[62] Some studies suggest that it is more cost-effective to initiate donepezil treatment in the milder stages of disease development and economic data support the use of both the 5 and 10 mg dosage regimens.[62]

Donepezil reduces nursing home costs by delaying the time before nursing-home placement becomes necessary.

Key points

- Donepezil is a reversible <u>acetylcholinesterase inhibitor</u> indicated for the symptomatic relief of mild-to-moderately severe Alzheimer's disease.

- Highly selective for <u>acetylcholinesterase</u> over <u>butyrylcholinesterase</u>, donepezil is most active in the central nervous system.

- Donepezil improves <u>cognitive</u> performance in a number of animal models of <u>cholinergic</u> deficiency and maintains regional brain glucose <u>metabolism</u> in patients with Alzheimer's disease.

- With a prolonged half life of 70–80 hours, donepezil can be administered once daily, in contrast to other agents of its class.

- The relatively slow <u>absorption</u> of donepezil limits the severity of cholinergic side-effects experienced by some patients.

- Donepezil has not been associated with any clinically significant <u>drug–drug interactions</u> and can be administered concomitantly with a variety of medications, with the possible exception of some compounds metabolised by the CYP enzymes.

- There is a significant correlation between the plasma concentration of donepezil and the extent of acetylcholinesterase inhibition, which plateaus at 76–84%. <u>ADAS-cog</u> and MMSE scores are similarly correlated with plasma drug levels.

- In patients with mild-to-moderate Alzheimer's disease, donepezil has proven benefits across all domains of <u>efficacy</u> – cognition, behaviour and function.

- Cognitive improvements are sustained for up to 2 years following initiation of donepezil treatment.

- In general, donepezil has a superior <u>adverse event</u> profile and discontinuation rate when compared with the cholinesterase inhibitors galantamine and rivastigmine.

- The majority of side-effects associated with donepezil are mild in severity and relate to peripheral cholinergic over-stimulation.

Any reference made to guidance from the National Institute of Clinical Excellence (NICE) in the preceding section relates to guidelines published in 2001. As we go to press (March 2005), NICE has issued preliminary guidance that is currently under review and will be finalised and published later in 2005 (see Editor's note Pages xx and 127).

References

A list of the published evidence which has been reviewed in compiling the preceding section of *BESTMEDICINE*.

1 Jones R. Have cholinergic therapies reached their clinical boundary in Alzheimer's disease? *Int J Geriatr Psychiatry* 2003; **18**: S7–13.

2 Cummings J. Use of cholinesterase inhibitors in clinical practice: evidence-based recommendations. *Am J Geriatr Psychiatry* 2003; **11**: 131–45.

3 Shigeta M, Homma A. Donepezil for Alzheimer's disease: pharmacodynamic, pharmacokinetic, and clinical profiles. *CNS Drug Rev* 2001; **7**: 353–68.

4 Eisai. Aricept (donepezil hydrochloride): prescribing information. Teaneck, NJ, 2002.

5 Saxena A, Fedorko J, Vinayaka C *et al.* Aromatic amino-acid residues at the active and peripheral anionic sites control the binding of E2020 (Aricept) to cholinesterases. *Eur J Biochem* 2003; **270**: 4447–58.

6 Goldsmith D, Scott L. Donepezil: in vascular dementia. *Drugs Aging* 2003; **20**: 1127–36.

7 Kasa P, Papp H, Kasa PJ, Torok I. Donepezil dose-dependently inhibits acetylcholinesterase activity in various areas and in the presynaptic cholinergic and the postsynaptic cholinoceptive enzyme-positive structures in the human and rat brain. *Neuroscience* 2000; **101**: 89–100.

8 Jann M, Shirley K, Small G. Clinical pharmacokinetics and pharmacodynamics of cholinesterase inhibitors. *Clin Pharmacokinet* 2002; **41**: 719–39.

9 Liston D, Nielsen J, Villalobos A *et al.* Pharmacology of selective acetylcholinesterase inhibitors: implications for use in Alzheimer's disease. *Eur J Pharmacol* 2004; **486**: 9–17.

10 Tiseo P, Rogers S, Friedhoff L. Pharmacokinetic and pharmacodynamic profile of donepezil HCl following evening administration. *Br J Clin Pharmacol* 1998; **46**: 13–18.

11 Doody R. Update on Alzheimer drugs (Donepezil). *The Neurologist* 2003; **9**: 225–9.

12 Kosasa T, Kuriya Y, Matsui K, Yamanishi Y. Inhibitory effects of donepezil hydrochloride (E2020) on cholinesterase activity in brain and peripheral tissues of young and aged rats. *Eur J Pharmacol* 1999; **386**: 7–13.

13 Ogura H, Kosasa T, Kuriya Y, Yamanishi Y. Donepezil, a centrally acting acetylcholinesterase inhibitor, alleviates learning deficits in hypocholinergic models in rats. *Methods Find Exp Clin Pharmacol* 2000; **22**: 89–95.

14 Luine V, Mohan G, Tu Z, Efange S. Chromaproline and chromaperidine, nicotine agonists, and donepezil, cholinesterase inhibitor, enhance performance of memory tasks in ovariectomized rats. *Pharmacol Biochem Behav* 2002; **74**: 213–20.

15 Tune L, Tiseo P, Ieni J *et al.* Donepezil HCl (E2020) maintains functional brain activity in patients with Alzheimer disease: results of a 24-week, double-blind, placebo-controlled study. *Am J Geriatr Psychiatry* 2003; **11**: 169–77.

16 Krishnan K, Charles H, Doraiswamy P *et al.* Randomized, placebo-controlled trial of the effects of donepezil on neuronal markers and hippocampal volumes in Alzheimer's disease. *Am J Psychiatry* 2003; **160**: 2003–11.

17 Thomas A, Iacono D, Bonanni L, D'Andreamatteo G, Onofrj M. Donepezil, rivastigmine, and vitamin E in Alzheimer disease: a combined P300 event-related potentials/neuropsychologic evaluation over 6 months. *Clin Neuropharmacol* 2001; **24**: 31–42.

18 Imbimbo B. Pharmacodynamic-tolerability relationships of cholinesterase inhibitors for Alzheimer's disease. *CNS Drugs* 2001; **15**: 375–90.

19 Rogers S, Friedhoff L. Pharmacokinetic and pharmacodynamic profile of donepezil HCl following single oral doses. *Br J Clin Pharmacol* 1998; **46**: 1–6.

20 Rogers S, Cooper N, Sukovaty R *et al.* Pharmacokinetic and pharmacodynamic profile of donepezil HCl following multiple oral doses. *Br J Clin Pharmacol* 1998; **46**: 7–12.

21 Hogan D, Patterson C. Progress in clinical neurosciences: Treatment of Alzheimer's disease and other dementias – review and comparison of the cholinesterase inhibitors. *Can J Neurol Sci* 2002; **29**: 306–14.

22 Tiseo P, Perdomo C, Friedhoff L. Metabolism and elimination of 14C-donepezil in healthy volunteers: a single-dose study. *Br J Clin Pharmacol* 1998; **46**: 19–24.

23 Tiseo P, Foley K, Friedhoff L. An evaluation of the pharmacokinetics of donepezil HCl in patients with moderately to severely impaired renal function. *Br J Clin Pharmacol* 1998; **46**: 56–60.

24 Tiseo P, Vargas R, Perdomo C, Friedhoff L. An evaluation of the pharmacokinetics of donepezil HCl in patients with impaired hepatic function. *Br J Clin Pharmacol* 1998; **46**: 51–5.

25 Rogers S, Friedhoff L. The efficacy and safety of donepezil in patients with Alzheimer's disease: results of a US multicentre, randomized, double-blind, placebo-controlled trial. The Donepezil Study Group. *Dementia* 1996; **7**: 293–303.

26 Rogers S, Doody R, Pratt R, Ieni J. Long-term efficacy and safety of donepezil in the treatment of Alzheimer's disease: final analysis of a US multicentre open-label study. *Eur Neuropsychopharmacol* 2000; **10**: 195–203.

27 Rogers S, Doody R, Mohs R, Friedhoff L. Donepezil improves cognition and global function in Alzheimer disease: a 15-week, double-blind, placebo-controlled study. Donepezil Study Group. *Arch Inter Med* 1998; **158**: 1021–31.

28 Rogers S, Farlow M, Doody R, Mohs R, Friedhoff L. A 24-week, double-blind, placebo-controlled trial of donepezil in patients with Alzheimer's disease. Donepezil Study Group. *Neurology* 1998; **50**: 136–45.

29 Burns A, Rossor M, Hecker J *et al.* The effects of donepezil in Alzheimer's disease – results from a multinational trial. *Dement Geriatr Cogn Disord* 1999; **10**: 237–44.

30 Gauthier S, Feldman H, Hecker J *et al.* Functional, cognitive and behavioral effects of donepezil in patients with moderate Alzheimer's disease. *Curr Med Res Opin* 2002; **18**: 347–54.

31 Homma A, Takeda M, Imai Y *et al.* Clinical efficacy and safety of donepezil on cognitive and global function in patients with Alzheimer's disease. A 24-week, multicenter, double-blind, placebo-controlled study in Japan. E2020 Study Group. *Dement Geriatr Cogn Disord* 2000; **11**: 299–313.

32 Tariot P, Cummings J, Katz I *et al.* A randomized, double-blind, placebo-controlled study of the efficacy and safety of donepezil in patients with Alzheimer's disease in the nursing home setting. *J Am Geriatr Soc* 2001; **49**: 1590–9.

33 Winblad B, Engedal K, Soininen H *et al.* A 1-year, randomized, placebo-controlled study of donepezil in patients with mild to moderate AD. *Neurology* 2001; **57**: 489–95.

34 Mohs R, Doody R, Morris J *et al.* A 1-year, placebo-controlled preservation of function survival study of donepezil in AD patients. *Neurology* 2001; **57**: 481–8.

35 Courtney C, Farrell D, Gray R *et al.* Long-term donepezil treatment in 565 patients with Alzheimer's disease (AD2000): randomised double-blind trial. *Lancet* 2004; **363**: 2105–15.

36 Doody R, Geldmacher D, Gordon B, Perdomo C, Pratt R. Open-label, multicenter, phase 3 extension study of the safety and efficacy of donepezil in patients with Alzheimer disease. *Arch Neurol* 2001; **58**: 427–33.

37 Nunez M, Jakab G, Jakobsen S, Johannsen P. Donepezil-treated Alzheimer's disease patients initially rated as showing 'no apparent clinical benefit' demonstrate significant benefits when therapy is continued. *American Geriatrics Society Annual Meeting 2003*: S99 Abstract.

38 Whitehead A, Perdomo C, Pratt R *et al.* Donepezil for the symptomatic treatment of patients with mild to moderate Alzheimer's disease: a meta-analysis of individual patient data from randomised controlled trials. *Int J Geriatr Psychiatry* 2004; **19**: 624–33.

39 Jones R, Soininen H, Hager K *et al.* A multinational, randomised, 12-week study comparing the effects of donepezil and galantamine in patients with mild to moderate Alzheimer's disease. *Int J Geriatr Psychiatry* 2004; **19**: 58–67.

40 Wilcock G, Howe I, Coles H *et al.* A long-term comparison of galantamine and donepezil in the treatment of Alzheimer's disease. *Drugs Aging* 2003; **20**: 777–89.

41 Wilkinson D, Passmore A, Bullock R *et al.* A multinational, randomised, 12-week, comparative study of donepezil and rivastigmine in patients with mild to moderate Alzheimer's disease. *Int J Clin Pract* 2002; **56**: 441–6.

42 Boada-Rovira M, Brodaty H, Cras P *et al.* Efficacy and safety of donepezil in patients with Alzheimer's disease: results of a global, multinational, clinical experience study. *Drugs Aging* 2004; **21**: 43–53.

43 Relkin N, Reichman W, Orazem J, McRae T. A large, community-based, open-label trial of donepezil in the treatment of Alzheimer's disease. *Dement Geriatr Cogn Disord* 2003; **16**: 15–24.

44 Hager K, Calabrese P, Frolich L, Gobel C, Berger F. An observational clinical study of the efficacy and tolerability of donepezil in the treatment of Alzheimer's disease. *Dement Geriatr Cogn Disord* 2003; **15**: 189–98.

45 Matthews H, Korbey J, Wilkinson D, Rowden J. Donepezil in Alzheimer's disease: eighteen month results from Southampton Memory Clinic. *Int J Geriatr Psychiatry* 2000; **15**: 713–20.

46 Froelich L, Gertz H, Heun R *et al.* Donepezil for Alzheimer's disease in clinical practice – The DONALD Study. A multicentre 24-week clinical trial in Germany. *Dement Geriatr Cogn Disord* 2004; **18**: 37–43.

47 Pedone C, Lapane K, Mor V, Bernabei R. Donepezil use in US nursing homes. *Aging Clin Exp Res.* 2004; **16**: 60–7.

48 Geldmacher D, Provenzano G, McRae T, Mastey V, Ieni J. Donepezil is associated with delayed nursing home placement in patients with Alzheimer's disease. *J Am Geriatr Soc* 2003; **51**: 937–44.

49 Lopez O, Becker J, Wisniewski S *et al.* Cholinesterase inhibitor treatment alters the natural history of Alzheimer's disease. *J Neurol Neurosurg Psychiatry* 2002; **72**: 310–14.

50 Fillit H, Gutterman E, Brooks R. Impact of donepezil on caregiving burden for patients with Alzheimer's disease. *Int Psychogeriatr* 2000; **12**: 389–401.

51 Wimo A, Winblad B, Engedal K *et al.* An economic evaluation of donepezil in mild to moderate Alzheimer's disease: results of a 1-year, double-blind, randomized trial. *Dement Geriatr Cogn Disord* 2003; **15**: 44–54.

52 Frolich L, Klinger T, Berger F. Treatment with donepezil in Alzheimer patients with and without cerebrovascular disease. *J Neurol Sci* 2002; **203–204**: 137–9.

53 Prasher V, Huxley A, Haque M. Down Syndrome Ageing Study Group. A 24-week, double-blind, placebo-controlled trial of donepezil in patients with Down syndrome and Alzheimer's disease – pilot study. *Int J Geriatr Psychiatry* 2002; **17**: 270–8.

54 Prasher V, Adams C, Holder R. Down Syndrome Research Group. Long term safety and efficacy of donepezil in the treatment of dementia in Alzheimer's disease in adults with Down syndrome: open label study. *Int J Geriatr Psychiatry* 2003; **18**: 549–51.

55 Doody R. Therapeutic standards in Alzheimer disease. *Alzheimer Dis Assoc Disord* 1999; **13**: S20–6.

56 Pratt R, Perdomo C, Surick I, Ieni J. Donepezil: tolerability and safety in Alzheimer's disease. *Int J Clin Pract* 2002; **56**: 710–17.

57 Dunn N, Pearce G, Shakir S. Adverse effects associated with the use of donepezil in general practice in England. *J Psychopharmacol* 2000; **14**: 406–8.

58 DeLaGarza V. Pharmacologic treatment of Alzheimer's disease: an update. *Am Fam Physician* 2003; **68**: 1365–72.

59 Clegg A, Bryant J, Nicholson T *et al*. Clinical and cost-effectiveness of donepezil, rivastigmine, and galantamine for Alzheimer's disease. A systematic review. *Int J Technol Assess Health Care* 2002; **18**: 497–507.

60 Wolfson C, Oremus M, Shukla V *et al*. Donepezil and rivastigmine in the treatment of Alzheimer's disease: a best-evidence synthesis of the published data on their efficacy and cost-effectiveness. *Clin Ther* 2002; **24**: 862–86.

61 Stewart A, Phillips R, Dempsey G. Pharmacotherapy for people with Alzheimer's disease: a Markov-cycle evaluation of five years' therapy using donepezil. *Int J Geriatr Psychiatry* 1998; **13**: 445–53.

62 Foster R, Plosker G. Donepezil. Pharmacoeconomic implications of therapy. *Pharmacoeconomics* 1999; **16**: 99–114.

63 Small G, Donohue J, Brooks R. An economic evaluation of donepezil in the treatment of Alzheimer's disease. *Clin Ther* 1998; **20**: 838–50.

Acknowledgements

Figure 2 is adapted from Tune *et al.*, 2003.[15]

Figure 3 is adapted from Rogers and Friedhoff, 1996.[25]

Figure 4 is adapted from Mohs *et al.*, 2001.[34]

Figure 5 is adapted from Whitehead *et al.*, 2001.[38]

Figure 6 is adapted from Jones *et al.*, 2004.[39]

3. Drug review – Galantamine (Reminyl®)

Dr Rebecca Fox-Spencer
CSF Medical Communications Ltd

Summary

Galantamine is the most recently introduced acetylcholinesterase inhibitor and is licensed in the UK for the treatment of mild-to-moderately severe Alzheimer's disease. Galantamine has a unique dual mechanism of action: in addition to raising the concentration of acetylcholine in the synaptic cleft, galantamine also acts directly on nicotinic acetylcholine receptors to increase both their sensitivity to acetylcholine and also may increase their number. These combined actions act to reduce the cholinergic deficit associated with Alzheimer's disease and have been shown to translate to significant clinical benefit relative to placebo. Thus, in large, placebo-controlled studies, galantamine was shown to reduce cognitive impairment, behavioural symptoms and caregiver burden, together with improving the ability to perform activities of daily living. In addition, galantamine is effective in reducing the incidence of behavioural symptoms associated with Alzheimer's disease. The safety and tolerability profile of galantamine is generally good, with an adverse event profile similar to that of other currently available acetylcholinesterase inhibitors. Adverse events associated with galantamine use are generally gastrointestinal in nature and mild-to-moderate in severity. They occur primarily during the dose-escalation phase of treatment, and can be minimised by ensuring that the dose is gradually increased and appropriately monitored.

You are strongly urged to consult your doctor before taking, stopping or changing any of the products reviewed or referred to in BESTMEDICINE or any other medication that has been prescribed or recommended by your doctor.

Introduction

Given the clearly established association between dementia in Alzheimer's disease and deficits in cholinergic neurotransmission within the cortex and hippocampus, it is not surprising that currently available treatments for Alzheimer's disease focus on restoring cholinergic function. These drugs act by inhibiting acetylcholinesterase, the enzyme responsible for the breakdown of the neurotransmitter acetylcholine to

Currently available treatments for Alzheimer's disease focus on restoring cholinergic function.

acetate and choline. The resulting treatment-related increases in concentrations of acetylcholine in the synaptic cleft are associated with significant improvements in cognitive ability in patients with Alzheimer's disease.[1,2]

The first generation of acetylcholinesterase inhibitors consisted of tacrine, velnacrine and physostigmine.[3] Whilst evidence from clinical trials showed that these drugs provided some clinical benefit, only tacrine was approved and its use was limited by its safety profile, particularly relating to hepatic toxicity and frequency of dosing.[4] A second generation of acetylcholinesterase inhibitors has superseded these agents, each of which lays claim to an improved tolerability profile, along with an increased specificity for acetylcholinesterase and/or an additional mode of action, compared with their predecessors.

Galantamine is the most recently introduced member of this group of drugs, despite being in clinical use for over 30 years as an anticurare agent to reverse muscle paralysis in anaesthesia. Galantamine is unique within this class in that it does not act solely through the inhibition of cholinesterase activity. In addition to its recognised inhibitory effects upon the acetylcholinesterase enzyme, galantamine exerts a modulating effect on nicotinic acetylcholine receptors, thereby increasing the intrinsic action of acetylcholine at these sites. These combined effects ensure good clinical efficacy in the treatment of mild-to-moderate Alzheimer's disease. Moreover, it has been speculated that galantamine could represent an advance towards agents that are not only effective in terms of symptomatic relief but which may also slow the progression of Alzheimer's disease and postpone neurodegenerative changes.[5] This article reviews the pharmacological properties of galantamine, and the impact that its novel dual mechanism of action – acting both as an acetylcholinesterase inhibitor and as a direct modulator of nicotinic acetylcholine receptors – has on its clinical efficacy, safety and tolerability.

> In addition to its recognised inhibitory effects upon the acetylcholinesterase enzyme, galantamine exerts a modulating effect on nicotinic acetylcholine receptors.

Pharmacology

Chemistry

> ☛ The chemistry of galantamine is of essentially academic interest and most healthcare professionals will, like you, skip this section.

The chemical structure of galantamine is shown in Figure 1. It is a tertiary alkaloid, originally derived from bulbs of the *Amaryllidaceae* family of flowering plants, though now generated synthetically in the form of galantamine hydrobromide.[2,6]

Mechanism of action

The inhibition of acetylcholinesterase by galantamine is specific, reversible and, in contrast to donepezil, competitive.[6] By inhibiting the breakdown of acetylcholine, galantamine increases its concentration in the synaptic cleft, thus counteracting the cholinergic deficit that is associated with Alzheimer's disease. In addition to direct inhibition of the enzyme, galantamine also exerts a modulating effect on nicotinic receptors (Figure 2). This effect, induced by the allosteric binding of

Figure 1. Chemical structure of galantamine.

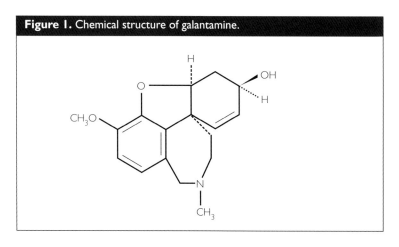

Figure 2. Mechanism of action of galantamine.[10]
ACh, acetylcholine; AChE, acetylcholinesterase; mAChR, muscarinic acetylcholine receptor;
nAchR, nicotinic acetylcholine receptor.

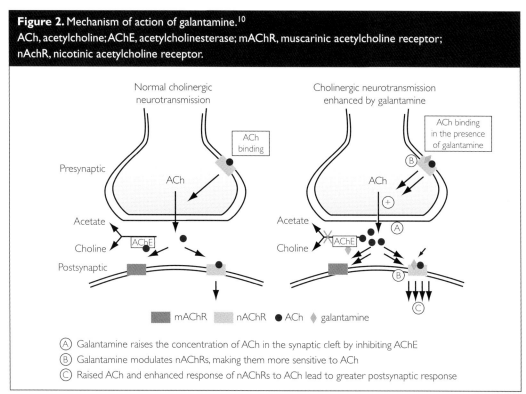

Normal cholinergic neurotransmission

Cholinergic neurotransmission enhanced by galantamine

ACh binding

ACh binding in the presence of galantamine

Presynaptic

ACh

ACh

Acetate

Choline

AChE

Postsynaptic

Acetate

Choline

AChE

■ mAChR ■ nAChR ● ACh ◆ galantamine

(A) Galantamine raises the concentration of ACh in the synaptic cleft by inhibiting AChE
(B) Galantamine modulates nAChRs, making them more sensitive to ACh
(C) Raised ACh and enhanced response of nAChRs to ACh lead to greater postsynaptic response

galantamine to this receptor (i.e. at a site distinct from the <u>acetylcholine</u> binding site), apparently increases the binding affinity of the receptor for acetylcholine and other acetylcholine agonists, as well as facilitating the conversion of the acetylcholine-bound receptor to its active state.[7] In this way, galantamine increases <u>cholinergic</u> activity in the central nervous system and reduces the impact of the cholinergic deficit that is apparent in patients with Alzheimer's disease.

In addition to its modulating effect upon <u>nicotinic receptors</u>, animal studies have indicated that long-term treatment with galantamine may be associated with increased numbers of these receptors in the hippocampus and neocortex.[8] Given that the loss of nicotinic receptors in patients with Alzheimer's disease correlates with the severity of disease at the time of the patient's death, this observation may account for an important therapeutic action of galantamine.[5] Indeed, there is evidence that selective loss of nicotinic receptors is the biochemical parameter that is most closely associated with the severity of Alzheimer's disease.[9]

Presynaptic nicotinic receptors can also modulate the release of other neurotransmitters, such as glutamate, serotonin and γ-aminobutyric acid.[10] These neurotransmitters are, in fact, more prominent players in the central nervous system than acetylcholine, and depletion of these may account for some of the psychotropic symptoms associated with Alzheimer's disease, such as attention deficits, aggression and sexual disinhibition.[10] Consequently, galantamine may afford further clinical benefits by indirectly modulating the levels of these neurotransmitters.

Preclinical studies

Inhibition of acetylcholinesterase

☛ *These preclinical data sections describe the results of the earliest phases of a drug's development (see Reader's Guide).*

In vitro studies have demonstrated that galantamine possesses a high degree of specificity for acetylcholinesterase. Thus, the concentration of galantamine required to inhibit the closely related (though less prevalent) enzyme, butyrylcholinesterase, is more than 50-times higher than that required to achieve the same magnitude of inhibition of acetylcholinesterase.[11] It has been suggested that dual inhibition of both enzymes is associated with an increased risk of necrotic damage, and that the specificity of galantamine for acetylcholinesterase may, therefore, lead to safety and tolerability benefits for patients.[11] However, in clinical trials, the adverse event profile and tolerability of galantamine is comparable with that of rivastigmine, which inhibits both enzymes.[12]

In human studies, a single 10 mg intravenous dose of galantamine administered to healthy volunteers was shown to generate a 65% inhibition of acetylcholinesterase within 2 minutes of administration. Oral doses of 5 or 10 mg galantamine administered to a patient with Alzheimer's disease generated a 50–70% inhibition of acetylcholinesterase within 2 hours of administration, with the effect being reversed within 2 hours of drug withdrawal.[11] A further study in eight healthy male volunteers demonstrated that intravenous administration of galantamine, 5 and 10 mg, inhibited acetylcholinesterase by 34 and 53%, respectively.[13]

Modulation of nicotinic receptors

A number of preclinical studies have evaluated galantamine's effects upon the nicotinic receptor. In one such study, a derivative of galantamine was introduced to cultured neuronal cell lines and was shown to have a potentiating effect on the response to acetylcholine.[7,9] This effect was independent of the degree of inhibition of acetylcholinesterase, and was related to a direct effect on the nicotinic receptor, as the same potentiating effect was observed when using agonists other than acetylcholine.[7] Moreover, the potentiating effect of galantamine was shown to be specific to nicotinic receptors, as galantamine did not alter the response of other receptors which bind acetylcholine, and whose inhibition may be associated with a more extensive side-effect profile. The potentiating effect of galantamine on nicotinic receptors, however, appears to be heavily dependent on its concentration; above a certain concentration threshold, this effect reverses and becomes inhibitory.[7]

Behavioural response to galantamine

Galantamine is less potent in terms of inhibition of the acetylcholinesterase enzyme than other currently available drugs in the class, such as donepezil and rivastigmine.[2,7] On this basis, galantamine might be expected to offer comparatively lower symptomatic control of dementia in patients with Alzheimer's disease. However, preliminary evidence from animal models indicates that galantamine is more effective than other acetylcholinesterase inhibitors in terms of behavioural responses.[14] This effect is most likely a consequence of galantamine's dual mechanism of action as additional efficacy is likely to be conferred by the direct effect of galantamine on the nicotinic receptors.

Studies using animal models of depleted cholinergic neurotransmission, which mimic the cholinergic deficit in patients with Alzheimer's disease, have demonstrated that galantamine can improve performance in spatial tasks of working memory.[15] However, galantamine appeared to impair performance in control animals without cholinergic deficits in this study. This was attributed to the use of relatively high concentrations of galantamine, which were sufficient to induce an inhibitory effect upon the nicotinic receptors as described previously.[15]

There are sparse preclinical data available that predict the effect of galantamine on human behaviour. In healthy elderly subjects, however, pharmacological modulation of nicotinic receptors using physostigmine and scopolamine has shown that this receptor is intrinsically involved in mediating arousal and selective attention.[16]

Pharmacokinetics

Absorption and distribution

The major pharmacokinetic parameters of galantamine in healthy male adults are summarised in Table 1.[5,10] Plasma clearance rates are reported to be 30–40% higher in patients with Alzheimer's disease than in young, healthy individuals.[17] The plasma clearance rate is also slightly greater in males than in females, though the difference is thought to be attributable to body weight, rather than gender *per se*.[17] Galantamine is rapidly absorbed following oral dosing, and has a shorter time (t_{max}) to peak plasma concentration (C_{max}) than donepezil, but is comparable with

☛ The *pharmacokinetics* of a drug are of interest to healthcare professionals because it is important for them to understand the action of a drug on the body over a period of time.

Table 1. The pharmacokinetic properties of galantamine following administration of a single oral 10 mg dose in healthy male volunteers.[5,10]

Pharmacokinetic parameter	
Absolute oral availability (%)	100
t_{max} (hours)	0.9–2.0
C_{max} (µg/L)	49–1150
Plasma protein binding (%)	18
$t_{1/2}$ (hours)	5–7
Plasma clearance (L/hour)	25
Volume of distribution (L)	175
AUC (µg.L/hour)	4770

AUC, area under the concentration–time curve; t_{max}, time to reach maximum plasma concentrations (C_{max}).

rivastigmine in this parameter.[18] The presence of food delays the absorption of galantamine (reducing C_{max} by approximately 25%) but has no impact on the overall extent of absorption, as represented by the AUC.[5] The pharmacokinetics of galantamine are linear with respect to plasma concentrations of the drug, when it is administered across the 4–16 mg dose range.[6] The large volume of distribution reflects the high degree of non-specific absorption of galantamine.[10] Bioavailability is very high and plasma protein binding low. Crucial to its role in treating Alzheimer's disease, galantamine crosses the blood–brain barrier.

Metabolism and elimination

In humans with normal metabolic capacity, approximately 75% of an administered galantamine dose is metabolised in the liver by the cytochrome P450 (CYP) enzymes 2D6 and 3A4, with the remaining 25% being excreted unchanged in the urine.[17,19] Only one of the resulting major metabolites has any significant acetylcholinesterase inhibitory activity, with a reported potency three-times that of galantamine in erythrocytes, which increases to six-times in brain homogenate.[20] However, this metabolite is not detectable in clinically relevant amounts in plasma, possibly because of its rapid inactivation.[20]

Given that galantamine is extensively metabolised by the CYP system, there is an increased potential for drug–drug interactions when galantamine is co-administered with inhibitors or activators of this system, particularly those that interact with CYP2D6 and 3A4 enzymes. Accordingly, the bioavailability of galantamine is increased considerably when it is co-administered with paroxetine (a CYP2D6 inhibitor) and ketoconazole or erythromycin (both CYP3A4 inhibitors).[6]

Pharmacokinetics in special patient populations

Given that the liver is the site of galantamine metabolism, it is important to evaluate its pharmacokinetic behaviour in individuals with impaired hepatic function. The presence of mild-to-moderate hepatic impairment reportedly has no effect on the adverse event profile of galantamine, and only once the impairment reaches moderate severity does there appear to be any impact on its pharmacokinetic profile.[21] Thus, no dosage adjustment is necessary in cases of mild hepatic impairment, although care should be taken over the initial dose-escalation phase in such cases. The use of galantamine is contra-indicated in individuals with severe hepatic impairment due to a lack of data in this patient population. The impact of hepatic impairment on the pharmacokinetics of galantamine is reported to be comparable with that of donepezil, and more favourable than that of rivastigmine.[21]

Along with CYP-mediated metabolic pathways, renal excretion is also critically involved in the elimination of galantamine. Although renal insufficiency appears to have less impact on the pharmacokinetics of galantamine compared with hepatic impairment, there is a lack of data supporting the drug's safety in populations with impaired renal function.[17] For patients with creatinine clearance greater than 9 mL/minute, no dosage adjustment is required.[2,6] However, the use of galantamine is contra-indicated in patients whose renal function is severely impaired (creatinine clearance less than 9 ml/min).[22]

> The use of galantamine is contra-indicated in individuals with severe hepatic impairment.

> Galantamine is contra-indicated in patients whose renal function is severely impaired.

Clinical efficacy

The clinical benefits of antidementia drugs can be identified by monitoring basic cognitive and global function. Perhaps of more relevance to the patient, however, is the impact of treatment on behavioural patterns, their ability to carry out daily tasks and their quality of life. A number of investigational instruments are available to quantify improvements in all of these parameters within a clinical trial setting.[5] Cognitive ability can be 'measured on the Mini-Mental State Examination (MMSE) scale, which is scored out of 30, with higher scores representing better cognitive function. It is used to establish baseline severity of illness in patients who are to be included in clinical trials, but is not ideally suited to longitudinal assessment due to a lack of sensitivity and a vulnerability to learning effects with repeated assessment. In a trial setting, cognitive function is better assessed by the Alzheimer's Disease Assessment Scale-cognitive subscale (ADAS-cog), which is scored out of 70, with higher scores representing greater cognitive impairments. This review refers specifically to the 11-item version of this scale, unless stated otherwise. Behavioural disturbances and neuropsychiatric symptoms are assessed on the Neuropsychiatric Inventory (NPI), which is scored out of 120, with a higher score reflecting greater disturbance. There is also an NPI caregiver distress scale, scored out of 60. The patient's ability to undertake tasks of daily living can be quantified on the Disability Assessment in Dementia (DAD) scale, scored out of 46, with a higher score indicating better functioning. Alternatively, the Alzheimer's Disease Cooperative Study that includes the Activities of Daily Living inventory (ADCS/ADL) is also widely used. This scale is scored out of 78, with higher scores indicating better functioning. The Progressive Deterioration Score (PDS) determines the ability to carry out tasks of daily living based on the patient's quality of life. This is a visual scale, with higher scores indicating better functioning. Sleep quality can be measured on the Pittsburgh Sleep Quality Index (PSQI), which is scored out of 21 with higher scores indicating a poorer quality of sleep. The Clinician Interview-Based Impression of Change plus Caregiver Input (CIBIC-plus) scale encompasses the patient's global state, cognition, behaviour and ability to carry out activities of daily living. This, and the similar Clinician Global Impression of Change (CGIC) scale are scored between 1 and 7, with higher scores indicating more marked deterioration. Similarly, the Nurses' Observation Scale for Geriatric Patients (NOSGER) combines scores for memory, instrumental activities of daily living, self-care, mood, social behaviour and disturbing behaviour.[5]

These scales, whilst providing a means to quantitate the efficacy of an antidementia drug, are subject to considerable inaccuracy due to their subjective nature. Furthermore, their relevance to real-life functional changes is questionable, and these limitations should be borne in mind when interpreting data from clinical trials.

Dose-ranging studies

Dose-ranging studies are particularly important to ensure that the optimum dose of a drug can be determined in order that benefit can be realised with the least risk of side-effects.

The efficacy and tolerability of a range of galantamine doses to treat patients with probable mild-to-moderate Alzheimer's disease (n=206) has been evaluated in a randomised, parallel-group, double-blind, placebo-controlled trial.[23] Following a 2-week wash-out phase, this 12-week trial incorporated a dose-escalation phase, to ultimate target doses of 18, 24 and 36 mg/day.

Interestingly, the middle galantamine dose (24 mg/day) generated the greatest average improvement in the ADAS-cog score relative to baseline (–1.4, compared with –0.1 and –0.7 for the lower and higher doses, respectively). Moreover, treatment with galantamine, 24 mg/day, provided the only statistically significant difference on ADAS-cog relative to placebo (mean change from baseline with placebo +1.6; $p=0.01$). Galantamine treatment was also associated with significant improvement compared with placebo on the PDS with the 24 mg/day dose ($p<0.05$), and on the CGI with the 32 mg/day dose ($p<0.05$). Adverse events occurred predominantly during the dose-escalation phase, and were generally mild and transient. The nature of these adverse events were similar to those reported with other acetylcholinesterase inhibitors, and included side-effects such as nausea and headache. Following the dose-escalation phase, the incidence of side-effects in actively treated patients declined to a level similar to that seen in the placebo group.

Thus, in conclusion, a 24 mg daily dose of galantamine appears to be the optimum dose to treat patients with mild-to-moderate Alzheimer's disease.[23] This observation is consistent with current treatment guidelines, which recommend dose escalation to a galantamine maintenance dose of 8–12 mg, administered twice daily.[22]

Placebo-controlled studies

Four large multicentre, placebo-controlled, randomised trials have evaluated the efficacy of galantamine in terms of cognitive ability in patients with probable mild-to-moderate Alzheimer's disease. Data from these studies are summarised in Table 2.[24–27] Two studies were conducted in the US,[25,27] whilst the other two were international.[24,26] All four placebo-controlled trials made similar evaluations of cognitive benefits, overall clinical response, impact on activities of daily living and the adverse event profile of galantamine. Two of these studies also generated additional data with regard to potential benefits on behavioural symptoms of dementia.[25,26]

Each study demonstrated significant benefits of galantamine treatment compared with placebo on the ADAS-cog. Treatment with galantamine, 24 and 32 mg/day, consistently demonstrated significantly better responses in terms of cognition than placebo (Figure 3). One of these studies demonstrated that 16 and 24 mg daily doses were effective in terms of cognitive improvement (–1.4 on ADAS-cog for both), whilst the 8 mg dose (+0.4) afforded no significant advantage over placebo (+1.7).[25] As well as providing improvements in terms of ADAS-cog score, galantamine treatment was also associated with a greater 'responder rate' (defined as an improvement of ≥4 points) on this scale than placebo across all four placebo-controlled studies.

The overall clinical response as determined by the CIBIC-plus scale was consistently improved with galantamine treatment at doses of 16, 24 and 32 mg/day, but not with the 8 mg daily dose or placebo.[24–27]

Galantamine treatment with 24 and 32 mg/day was shown to improve the ability to carry out activities of daily living compared with placebo as determined by the DAD scale and the ADCS/ADL.[24–26] However, one study failed to detect any significant deviation from baseline in DAD score after 6 months' treatment with either placebo or galantamine.[27] Following the 6-month open-label extension phase of this study, the group who had received placebo during the double-blind phase demonstrated a significant decline from baseline in DAD score (mean decrease of 8.1), whereas galantamine treatment maintained the ability of patients to carry out activities of daily living (mean decrease of 1.7).[27]

The two studies which evaluated the effect of galantamine treatment on behavioural and psychological symptoms of Alzheimer's disease quantified the benefits according to the NPI, which assesses ten domains of behavioural symptoms.[25,26] One 5-month study demonstrated a significant benefit of galantamine treatment compared with placebo in terms of NPI score over this time frame. Thus, NPI scores were maintained at baseline in the galantamine group but declined in those receiving placebo.[25] The more recently conducted of the two studies

Current treatment guidelines recommend dose escalation to a galantamine maintenance dose of 8–12 mg, twice daily.

Table 2. Summary of multicentre, double-blind, randomised, placebo-controlled trials evaluating galantamine for the treatment of mild-to-moderate Alzheimer's disease.[24–27] Statistical relationships are reported according to intention-to-treat analyses in preference to per-protocol analyses.

Study	Study design	Main outcomes
Wilcock et al., 2000[24]	6 months following 4-week run-in phase (n=653) Galantamine, 24 or 32 mg/day, or placebo	• At 6 months, the mean change from baseline in ADAS-cog score was –0.5 and –0.8 for galantamine 24 and 32 mg/day respectively, with both doses significantly superior to placebo (score of +2.4; $p<0.001$). The greatest benefit on ADAS-cog was for patients with moderately severe disease. • Both doses of galantamine improved outcome on CIBIC-plus ratings at 6 months ($p<0.05$ vs placebo for 24 mg/day, $p<0.001$ for 32 mg/day). • Galantamine treatment was associated with less decline in DAD scores after 6 months' treatment (–3.2 and –2.5 for 24 and 32 mg/day respectively), than was observed in the placebo-treated group (–6.0). The benefit on this scale of 32 mg/day galantamine over placebo was significant ($p<0.05$). • Some adverse events occurred more frequently following galantamine treatment than with placebo. Most were mild-to-moderate and gastrointestinal. Weight loss was slightly more common in galantamine-treated patients (occurring in 8% of those receiving 24 mg/day and 5% of those receiving 32 mg/day) than in the placebo group (0.5%). • Discontinuations due to adverse events were more frequent amongst galantamine-treated patients (22% in 24 mg/day group and 14% in 32 mg/day group) than placebo (9%). Approximately half of these discontinuations occurred during the dose-escalation phase.
Tariot et al., 2000[25]	5 months following 4-week run-in phase (n=978) Galantamine, 8, 16, or 24 mg/day, or placebo	• The mean change from baseline in ADAS-cog was –1.4 for the two higher doses of galantamine, and +0.4 in the lowest dose group. Galantamine at 16 and 32 mg/day was statistically superior to placebo (+1.7; $p<0.001$), but the 8 mg dose provided no significant advantage over placebo. • Improvements in ADAS-cog scores compared with baseline were significantly greater with the 16 or 24 mg daily doses than with the 8 mg dose ($p<0.05$ and $p<0.01$, respectively). • Galantamine, 16 and 24 mg/day, produce significantly greater improvements in CIBIC-plus scores than the 8 mg dose ($p<0.05$) and placebo ($p<0.001$).

ADAS-cog, Alzheimer's Disease Assessment Scale-cognitive subscale; ADCS/ADL, Alzheimer's disease Cooperative Study that includes Activities of Daily Living; CIBIC-plus, Clinician Interview-Based Impression of Change plus Caregiver Input; DAD, Disability Assessment in Dementia; NPI, Neuropsychiatric Inventory; PSQI, Pittsburgh Sleep Quality Index.

Table 2. Continued

Study	Study design	Main outcomes
		• Significantly smaller decreases in ADCS/ADL score were reported with galantamine, 16 and 24 mg/day (–0.7 and –1.5, respectively), than with placebo (–3.8; $p<0.01$). The decrease in ADCS/ADL score with galantamine at 8 mg/day was –3.2, which was significantly inferior to 16 mg/day, but not the 24 mg/day dose ($p<0.01$). Only the 16 mg/day dose yielded an ADCS/ADL score at study endpoint which was not significantly deteriorated from baseline.
		• Galantamine at 16 and 24 mg/day prevented deterioration of NPI score (mean change from baseline –0.1 and 0.0, respectively), affording significant benefit over placebo (mean change of +2.0; $p<0.05$). Galantamine at 8 mg/day, however, was associated with significant deterioration from baseline (+2.3; $p<0.05$).
		• A number of adverse events occurred more frequently following galantamine than placebo treatment, though most were mild in severity. A slight dose-related weight loss was reported in galantamine-treated patients. The rate of treatment discontinuation due to adverse events was similar in galantamine-treated patients and the placebo group.
		• There were no clinically relevant differences in safety measures.
Rockwood et al., 2001[26]	3 months following 4-week run-in phase (n=386) Galantamine, 24 or 32 mg/day, or placebo	• There were significant cognitive benefits associated with galantamine treatment (data from both doses combined) according to ADAS-cog scores at 3 months (mean change from baseline –0.9 with galantamine vs +0.7 with placebo; $p<0.01$). There were no significant differences between doses.
		• Significant global responses according to the CIBIC-plus scale at 3 months were reported with galantamine treatment (both doses combined; $p<0.01$ vs placebo).
		• The mean deterioration from baseline over 3 months with galantamine (both doses combined) of –1.2 on the DAD scale was significantly less than that seen with placebo (–5.3, $p<0.01$).
		• There was no significant difference in the mean change from baseline in NPI scores following 3 months of galantamine (–0.4) or placebo (+0.5) treatment.
		• Some adverse events occurred more often following galantamine than placebo treatment, mostly mild-to-moderate in severity.

ADAS-cog, Alzheimer's Disease Assessment Scale-cognitive subscale; ADCS/ADL, Alzheimer's disease Cooperative Study that includes Activities of Daily Living; CIBIC-plus, Clinician Interview-Based Impression of Change plus Caregiver Input; DAD, Disability Assessment in Dementia; NPI, Neuropsychiatric Inventory; PSQI, Pittsburgh Sleep Quality Index.

Table 2. Continued

Study	Study design	Main outcomes
		• There were no changes from baseline in PSQI scores after 3 months' treatment with galantamine or placebo (mean decrease of 0.2 points in each case).
		• There were no clinically relevant differences in safety measures.
Raskind et al., 2000[27]	6 months following 4-week run-in phase (n=636)	• After 6 months, both doses of galantamine improved scores on ADAS-cog (−1.9 and −1.4 for 24 and 32 mg/day, respectively) and were statistically superior to placebo, which was associated with cognitive decline (+2.0; $p<0.001$ vs placebo for both doses).
	6-month, open-label extension (galantamine, 24 mg/day) (n=353)	• Both doses of galantamine led to a better outcome on CIBIC-plus ratings than placebo at both 3 and 6 months ($p<0.05$ for all comparisons).
	Galantamine, 24 or 32 mg/day, or placebo	• There was no significant deviation in DAD scores from baseline in any group at 6 months. There was a significant decline at 12 months in the group who had received placebo during the double-blind phase (−8.1), but no significant decrease relative to baseline associated with galantamine treatment(24 mg/day) (−1.7).
		• Some adverse events occurred more frequently following galantamine treatment than with placebo. These were mostly mild-to-moderate in severity and gastrointestinal in nature. A slight weight loss reported in the double-blind phase was restored during the extension phase.
		• Discontinuations due to adverse events were more common in galantamine-treated subjects (23% in 24 mg/day group, 32% in 32 mg/day group) than in the placebo group (8%). These occurred mostly during the dose-escalation phase.

ADAS-cog, Alzheimer's Disease Assessment Scale-cognitive subscale; ADCS/ADL, Alzheimer's disease Cooperative Study that includes Activities of Daily Living; CIBIC-plus, Clinician Interview-Based Impression of Change plus Caregiver Input; DAD, Disability Assessment in Dementia; NPI, Neuropsychiatric Inventory; PSQI, Pittsburgh Sleep Quality Index.

failed to demonstrate any significant deviation of NPI scores from baseline with either active or placebo treatment, but this assessment was made after only 3 months of the study.[26]

All four placebo-controlled studies recorded patients' experiences of adverse events, and identified those side-effects which occurred at least 5% more often in the galantamine group than in the placebo group. Consistent with the dose-ranging study described previously, adverse events were generally mild-to-moderate in severity and most frequent during the dose-escalation phase. These side-effects tended to be gastrointestinal in nature and included nausea, vomiting and diarrhoea. Galantamine treatment was also associated with anorexia and weight

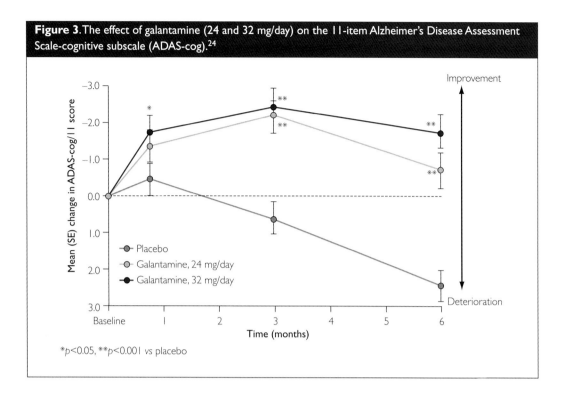

Figure 3. The effect of galantamine (24 and 32 mg/day) on the 11-item Alzheimer's Disease Assessment Scale-cognitive subscale (ADAS-cog).[24]

*p<0.05, **p<0.001 vs placebo

loss, though in the study that included an open-label extension phase, weight loss was partially reversed with continuing treatment.[27] Given the anticurare property of galantamine, three of the trials specifically evaluated the incidence of muscle weakness following treatment.[25–27] Such events were considered to be rare and were no more likely to occur with galantamine, 8–32 mg/day, than with placebo. Reports have shown that acetylcholinesterase inhibitors may be associated with sleep disturbances.[28] However, following 3 months of galantamine treatment (24 or 32 mg/day) no significant changes in sleep quality were reported, as assessed by the Pittsburgh sleep quality index (PSQI).[26]

Post hoc analyses

Data from the 5-month US study has subsequently undergone secondary analyses, which focused on the functional and behavioural implications of galantamine therapy.[29,30] Whereas the original study primarily focused on cognitive function, these two subsequent analyses have considered the more clinically relevant outcomes of ability to perform activities of daily living and caregiver burden. It has been hypothesised that cognitive and behavioural responses to a drug may dissociate, since they are mediated by different regions in the brain.[29] The first *post hoc* analysis demonstrated that galantamine-treated patients showed significantly less aberrant motor behaviour, apathy and disinhibition over the course of the study than those who received placebo.[29] In those patients with behavioural abnormalities at baseline,

Galantamine-treated patients showed significantly less aberrant motor behaviour, apathy and disinhibition over the course of the study than those who received placebo.

galantamine reduced scores for aberrant motor behaviour, agitation and anxiety by 29–48%. Behaviour-related caregiver distress was significantly reduced amongst the caregivers of patients who received galantamine, 24 mg/day. In terms of behavioural symptoms, the NPI demonstrated that galantamine-treated patients had improved in terms of depression/dysphoria, disinhibition, hallucinations and irritability/lability. As caregiver distress is specifically linked to patient behaviour, it is likely that the observed improvements in behavioural symptoms were directly related to improvements in caregiver burden.

In a second *post hoc* analysis of the 5-month US study, improvements in the ability to perform activities of daily living (as determined by ADCS/ADL scores) were shown to correlate significantly with treatment-related improvements in cognitive function.[30] The greatest improvements in ADCS/ADL scores were reported in those patients with the most severe dementia at baseline, as defined by patients' MMSE scores. At the end of the study, galantamine-treated patients performed significantly better than the placebo group in a number of basic and 'instrumental' activities of daily living (Table 3).

Of the four pivotal placebo-controlled trials described in the preceding section, data from the two 6-month trials have also been subject to a *post hoc* analysis, in order to determine the effects of galantamine treatment on caregiver time.[31] Although the study investigators conceded that this parameter is subject to considerable error, they estimated that caregivers of patients treated with galantamine spend an average of 3.5 hours less per week assisting patients relative to those in the placebo group.

Data concerning treatment with galantamine (24 mg/day) across the placebo-controlled studies were also examined to determine whether the efficacy of galantamine extended to a subgroup of the patient population who were over the age of 80 years.[32] Patients in this 'older' population demonstrated significantly better cognitive function with galantamine than with placebo (mean difference of 2.9 points at 6 months; $p<0.01$). The cognitive benefit of galantamine relative to projected placebo data was maintained for at least 12 months (at which point the difference in

Table 3. Activities of daily living in which galantamine, 16 or 24 mg/day, was reported to be significantly more effective than placebo.[30]

Galantamine dose	Basic activities	Instrumental activities
16 mg/day	• Walking • Grooming	• Television • Managing personal belongings • Current events • Writing • Household appliances
24 mg/day	• Eating	• Current events • Writing

ADAS-cog score was 4.3; $p<0.01$). Significant benefits of galantamine over placebo were also observed in CIBIC-plus scores at 6 months. The tolerability profile of galantamine in this patient population was comparable with that seen in the study population as a whole. The study investigators commented that these results reinforce UK-based treatment guidelines which advise that acetylcholinesterase treatment should be made available to all patients with mild-to-moderate Alzheimer's disease, regardless of age. However, older age groups of patients are currently under-represented amongst the treated population in the UK.[32,33]

Comparative clinical trials

Donepezil is currently the most widely prescribed drug used to treat mild-to-moderate Alzheimer's disease and accounts for approximately 45% of prescriptions given to the treated Alzheimer's population in the US.[34]

A 12-month, head-to-head, rater-blinded, randomised clinical trial of galantamine and donepezil has been conducted in the UK.[35] Due to ethical reasons, no placebo arm was included in this study. In addition, since the two drugs have different dosing and dose-escalation schedules, the study was rater-blinded rather than double-blinded. Subjects were excluded if they were previous users of galantamine or donepezil, or had other neurodegenerative disorders or causes of cognitive impairment. A total of 94 patients were randomised to galantamine and 88 to donepezil. The only baseline difference of note between the two groups was an over-representation of females in the donepezil group. Patients in the galantamine group were initially given 4 mg twice daily, then 8 mg twice daily from week 5, increasing to 12 mg twice daily at week 13, at the discretion of the investigator. Similarly, donepezil was initially administered at 5 mg once daily, increasing to 10 mg once daily, at week 5.[35]

In this study, the primary outcome measure was the Bristol Activities of Daily Living Scale (BADLS), which is rated by the caregiver. A functional decline was observed on this scale in both groups from month 9 with no statistically significant differences apparent between the two treatment groups at study endpoint.[35] However, the authors of this report highlight that this was the first reported use of the BADLS in a long-term clinical study. As such, the sensitivity of this tool may be insufficient to detect differences between the treatment groups given the size of the study population.

The effect on cognition was a secondary outcome in this study. When considering the entire study population, there was a non-significant trend for superiority of galantamine in terms of effect on cognition compared with donepezil according to the ADAS-cog and the MMSE. However, when only data from the sub-population in whom treatment is indicated according to clinical guidelines (i.e. those with baseline MMSE score 12–18)[33] were considered, galantamine demonstrated statistically significant superiority over donepezil (Figure 4). Galantamine also demonstrated superior efficacy over

These results reinforce UK-based treatment guidelines which advise that acetylcholinesterase treatment should be made available to all patients with mild-to-moderate Alzheimer's disease, regardless of age.

Galantamine was superior in terms of effect on cognition compared with donepezil according to the ADAS-cog and the MMSE.

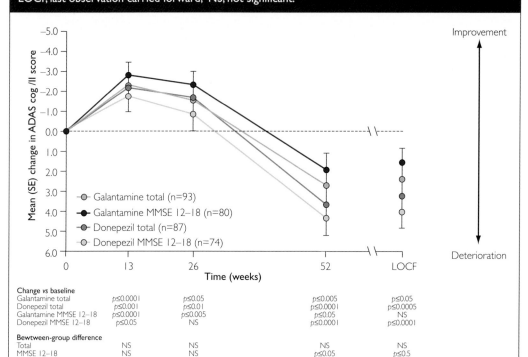

Figure 4. The effect of galantamine (16 or 24 mg/day) and donepezil (5 or 10 mg/day) on the 11-item Alzheimer's Disease Assessment Scale-cognitive subscale (ADAS-cog), in the total study population and in those with baseline Mini Mental State Examination (MMSE) scores of 12–18.[35]
LOCF, last observation carried forward; NS, not significant.

donepezil in terms of reducing caregiver burden, though no significant differences were reported in terms of NPI score for the two drugs.

A more recently conducted comparative study has also evaluated the relative efficacy and tolerability of galantamine and donepezil in a total of 120 patients with mild-to-moderate Alzheimer's disease.[36] This trial was open-label in design, and therefore not directly comparable with the rater-blinded trial described above. This randomised, multicentre trial was, nonetheless, similar in design to the aforementioned comparative study and employed the same dosing schedules. This trial was carried out over the considerably shorter period of 12 weeks. In contrast to the study of Wilcock *et al.*,[35] this trial demonstrated clear superiority for donepezil over galantamine in terms of satisfaction and ease of use, as evaluated by both physicians and caregivers. Donepezil also offered superior efficacy to galantamine in terms of cognition as determined by ADAS-cog (11 and 13 item scales) and MMSE scores and in activities of daily living as determined by the DAD. The investigators proposed that the lower efficacy of galantamine on these cognitive measures might be a consequence of a longer dose-escalation phase for galantamine than for donepezil, thereby exposing patients to the target maintenance dose of galantamine for a shorter duration of time.[36] Given that this study was only 12 weeks in duration, the additional 4 weeks spent in the dose-escalation phase may indeed have had some impact on overall efficacy. This was less likely to be the case during the Wilcock study, in which a 4-week delay in reaching target maintenance dose represents a considerably smaller proportion of the total study duration.

Although both treatments were well tolerated in this trial, galantamine was associated with a higher incidence of adverse events, with significantly more discontinuations as a consequence than was observed in the donepezil group.[36] Interestingly, significantly more patients receiving donepezil remained at the maximum dose at their last visit than those in the galantamine group. Consistent with this observation, more patients receiving galantamine made unscheduled visits to their physician due to dose tolerability problems than those who received donepezil.[36]

In terms of global response to treatment, a meta-analysis has indicated that donepezil offers superiority over galantamine.[3] However, a more recently conducted meta-analysis has indicated there is little basis to recommend one acetylcholinesterase inhibitor above any other in terms of cognitive or global benefit.[12] Unlike donepezil and rivastigmine, the benefits afforded by galantamine did not appear to be affected by its dose in this analysis. Although patients treated with galantamine were least likely to complete clinical trials, there was a dose-dependency of adverse events in these patients. As galantamine demonstrates good clinical efficacy at low–medium doses, problems with poorer tolerability at higher doses may be somewhat irrelevant in clinical practice.[3,12] Indeed, this meta-analysis reported that the risk of experiencing adverse events was similar for donepezil, 5 mg/day, and galantamine, 16–18 mg/day. Likewise, donepezil, 10 mg/day, and galantamine, 24 mg/day, had a similar risk of experiencing adverse events. Only those patients who received galantamine, 32–36 mg/day, which exceeds the licensed dose,[22] had a risk which clearly exceeded that seen in donepezil-treated patients.[12]

Despite these conflicting data, one may expect potential advantages of galantamine over donepezil or rivastigmine as a consequence of its additional modulating effect at nicotinic receptors. Rivastigmine also has a dual mode of action, inhibiting butyrylcholinesterase as well as acetylcholinesterase, though the lower prevalence of the former enzyme limits the potential impact of this property on the clinical efficacy of rivastigmine. The effect of galantamine on nicotinic receptors may be partially responsible for the reported sustained duration of efficacy of galantamine,[37,38] and is perhaps the most likely factor responsible for the benefits to behaviour and mood associated with galantamine treatment.[25,39] It should be noted, however, that there is a paucity of data from comparative clinical trials or meta-analyses concerning the relative psychotropic benefits of the various cholinesterase inhibitors.[29] The case for a specific psychotropic effect of galantamine is by no means strong, and appropriately designed longer-term studies are needed in order to determine whether the effect of galantamine on nicotinic receptors constitutes a neuroprotective effect.[12]

The effect of galantamine on nicotinic receptors is perhaps the most likely factor responsible for the benefits to behaviour and mood.

Efficacy in clinical practice

The populations studied in the clinical trials considered to date are subject to extensive inclusion and exclusion criteria. For example, patients with evidence of concomitant neurodegenerative disorders were excluded from entry into clinical studies,[24–27] as were those with any previous exposure to acetylcholinesterase inhibitors.[24,26] A number of open-label trials have now been conducted within a real-life, clinical practice setting, which apply a minimum of inclusion and exclusion criteria. Whilst these trials are not placebo-controlled, they do provide some preliminary evidence of how galantamine can be expected to perform in clinical practice in patients with probable mild-to-moderate Alzheimer's disease.

One such study recruited 36 patients, aged over 50 years, from the Belfast City Hospital Memory Clinic.[40] The only criteria for entry into this study were that concomitant medications for Alzheimer's disease were stable for 3 months prior to study entry, there were no contra-indications to acetylcholinesterase inhibitors and a caregiver was available to ensure patient compliance to treatment. Patients (mean age of 78 years) demonstrated significant improvements from baseline in cognitive ability, behavioural symptoms and behaviour-related caregiver distress following 3 months of galantamine treatment. Only caregiver distress levels remained significantly improved over baseline following 6 months of treatment. Galantamine was well tolerated in this study, with adverse events generally mild-to-moderate and gastrointestinal in nature. Thus, results from this small, open-label study are consistent with those from placebo-controlled trials.[40]

The benefits of galantamine treatment have also been demonstrated in naturalistic studies that have focused on the behavioural disturbances and neuropsychiatric symptoms associated with Alzheimer's disease – symptoms that are considered by many to be more clinically relevant than cognitive impairment.[41] A 3-month study of 124 community-dwelling out-patients attending hospital centres in Switzerland has demonstrated significant improvements in neuropsychiatric symptoms (mean change from baseline on NPI of –3.6) and caregiver burden (mean change from baseline on NPI caregiver distress scale of –1.9) with galantamine administered at 24 mg/day.[42] This study also reported improvements in physician- and nurse-rated observations (assessed on the CGI and NOSGER scales). A Brazilian open-label study of 33 patients demonstrated significant benefits of galantamine in terms of computerised neuropsychological tests of attention and memory.[43] Improvements were reported in reaction time, but not in the percentage of correct responses, which indicates that the benefits of galantamine were most marked in the domain of attention.[43] A drug-utilisation study in Italy showed a short-term, moderate cognitive benefit of acetylcholinesterase inhibitor treatment (galantamine, donepezil or rivastigmine), yet little gain in the ability of the patient to perform activities of daily living or in overall global functioning.[44] The authors suggested that the more 'complex' nature of the naturalistic population may account for this discrepancy with clinical trial data. It must be

Benefits of galantamine treatment have been demonstrated in naturalistic studies that have focused on the behavioural disturbances and neuropsychiatric symptoms associated with Alzheimer's disease.

considered, however, that the study population in this study was not randomised to drug treatment with the choice of drug being at the discretion of the physician. Indeed, only 5% of the population were treated with galantamine.[44]

Data applicable to the use of galantamine in clinical practice are also available from two open-label extensions of placebo-controlled trials.[37,38] Both extensions demonstrate sustained cognitive benefits associated with galantamine treatment (24 mg/day) according to ADAS-cog. When these data were combined with those from the original double-blind phases of the studies, the reported benefits of galantamine treatment, compared with the predicted cognitive decline of untreated patients, extended over durations of 18.5 and 36 months.[37,38]

Special patient populations

All of the drugs currently licensed for use in the UK for treatment of patients with mild-to-moderate Alzheimer's disease are acetylcholinesterase inhibitors. It is likely, therefore, that a significant proportion of patients that are prescribed galantamine may have a history of acetylcholinesterase inhibitor therapy. Some evidence suggests that benefits may be apparent when switching treatment from one acetylcholinesterase inhibitor to another.[34] A *post hoc* analysis of one of the placebo-controlled trials described above explored the effect of prior use of acetylcholinesterase inhibitors on the outcome of treatment with galantamine.[25,45] This analysis revealed no differences in terms of clinical efficacy or safety/tolerability, and therefore concluded that discontinuation of prior acetylcholinesterase inhibitor treatment does not preclude the possibility of future effective treatment with galantamine.[45]

Another patient population worthy of specific consideration includes those individuals with an over-representation of ε4 apolipoprotein alleles. The ApoE 4 genotype is a susceptibility factor for the earlier onset of Alzheimer's disease.[46] The first-generation acetylcholinesterase inhibitor tacrine demonstrated a reduced effect in ε4 carriers. As such, the ApoE 4 genotype was used as a predictor of response to tacrine therapy. Galantamine has been shown to elicit cognitive and functional improvement in over 1500 patients with Alzheimer's disease independently of their ε4 allele status.[46] The benefits of galantamine in this patient population were confirmed by data from two of the placebo-controlled clinical trials.[24,27]

It is beyond the scope of this review to discuss the efficacy of galantamine in patients with types of dementia which are not due to Alzheimer's disease. Nevertheless, it is worth considering that Alzheimer's disease and cerebrovascular factors that contribute to dementia, are not mutually exclusive. Data are available demonstrating that galantamine is effective and well tolerated in patients with probable vascular and 'mixed' dementia (i.e. Alzheimer's disease with cerebrovascular disease).[47]

> Discontinuation of prior acetylcholinesterase inhibitor treatment does not preclude the possibility of future effective treatment with galantamine.

Safety and tolerability

Treatment with galantamine is associated with a range of side-effects, the majority of which are consistent with those reported for other acetylcholinesterase inhibitors. Such adverse events are generally mild-to-moderate in severity and usually gastrointestinal in nature. Three of the four major placebo-controlled trials of galantamine that have been described in this review have reported adverse events that occur at least 5% more frequently in the treated group than in the placebo group, and have presented these data according to dose.[24,25,27] The cumulative findings of these three trials are shown in Figure 5.

Adverse events often subside following the initial dose-escalation phase.[24,27] Indeed, the dose-escalation phase appears to be critical in determining a patient's tolerance to the drug. Thus, to minimise the likelihood of adverse events, the manufacturer recommends that doses are increased no more abruptly than at 4-weekly increments.[25,34]

Patients with Alzheimer's disease are known to be at an increased risk of sleep-related problems, with increased levels of time awake at night and reduced amounts of rapid eye movement (REM) and slow-wave sleep.[28,48] These disturbances can exacerbate behavioural problems and are associated with increased stress levels amongst caregivers. It is noteworthy that donepezil treatment was reported to increase insomnia and abnormal dreams.[28] Insomnia is claimed as a common side-effect

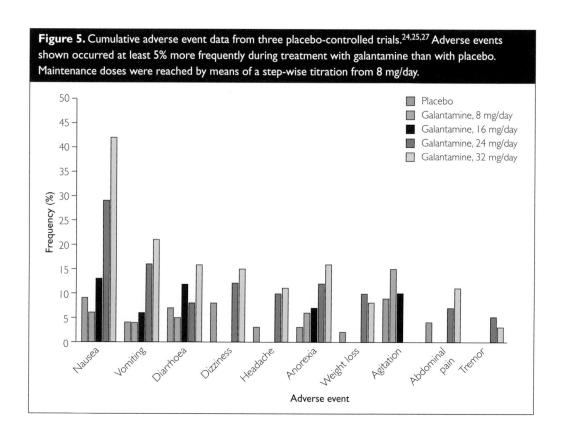

Figure 5. Cumulative adverse event data from three placebo-controlled trials.[24,25,27] Adverse events shown occurred at least 5% more frequently during treatment with galantamine than with placebo. Maintenance doses were reached by means of a step-wise titration from 8 mg/day.

associated with galantamine treatment, though data from clinical trials tend to report a neutral effect on sleep.[6,26,48]

As is the case with other drugs that act on the cholinergic system, caution is advised when galantamine is used in patients with a range of comorbid conditions. For example, in certain cardiovascular, gastrointestinal, neurological, pulmonary and genitourinary conditions, the use of galantamine should be subject to close monitoring.[6] Galantamine is not recommended in patients with gastrointestinal obstruction or those recovering from gastrointestinal surgery. Likewise, in patients with urinary outflow obstruction or those recovering from bladder surgery, the use of galantamine is not advised. Given the anticurare property of galantamine, it will also exaggerate muscle relaxation during anaesthesia.[6] As described earlier, the use of galantamine is contra-indicated in patients with severe hepatic failure due to its hepatic metabolism and the lack of data concerning its safety in this patient population.[21] Similarly, galantamine is contra-indicated in patients with severe renal failure.

Animal studies have indicated that galantamine treatment is associated with a slight delay in the development of the foetus or neonate. Clearly, pregnant or breast-feeding women do not constitute a significant proportion of the population with Alzheimer's disease. Nevertheless, galantamine is contra-indicated in these groups, as it is in children.[6] Galantamine has vagotonic effects on heart rate, and so should be used with caution in patients with sick sinus syndrome or other supra-ventricular cardiac conduction disturbances.[6]

In order to avoid drug–drug interactions, galantamine should not be co-administered with other cholinomimetics, and care should be taken if concomitant medication significantly reduces the heart rate.[6] As described previously, inhibitors of the CYP2D6 and CYP3A4 isoenzymes increase the bioavailability of galantamine, and therefore caution is advised when co-administering these agents with galantamine. Based on the tolerability response, a reduction in the maintenance dose of galantamine may be considered in such cases.[2,6]

Pharmacoeconomics

The cost of managing Alzheimer's disease increases with the severity of the disease, which reflects the transition of care from unpaid care, through paid care in the community, to institutionalisation. Evaluations of the impact which galantamine treatment has on these costs have relied on projection of data available from clinical trials to long-term anticipated outcomes using a theoretical model. The Assessment of Health Economics in Alzheimer's Disease (AHEAD) model has been used in a number of analyses in Europe and North America, including one study in the UK.[49,50] This model focuses on predicting at what point full-time care would be necessary, defining this state as a consistent requirement for a significant amount of care giving and supervision each day, regardless of the location or the identity of the caregiver.[51]

The UK study (using 2001 costs), applied the AHEAD model to data from three placebo-controlled clinical trials.[24,25,27,49] The model predicted that, without pharmacological intervention, the mean period of time until full-time care was necessary was 3.2 years, and the mean total survival time was 5.1 years. If treated with galantamine, the total time spent in full-time care was reduced by an average of 12% (with galantamine, 16 mg/day) or 15% (galantamine, 24 mg/day). Over the first 3 years, there was a net cost of treatment relative to no intervention. However, over a total of 10 years, it was estimated that 80% of the overall treatment cost would be offset by the financial benefits of delaying the need for full-time care. Over this period, the cost of care was estimated to be £28,134 in the absence of any pharmacological intervention, over two-thirds of which were attributable to the costs of providing full-time care. In order to delay the requirement for full-time care by 1 month, the net cost of treatment with galantamine, 16 mg/day, was estimated to be £192 per patient.[49]

Pharmacoeconomic modelling using the AHEAD model in other European countries and in the US has generated more favourable pharmacoeconomic estimates for the use of galantamine.[50,52] One study has reported that net cumulative costs become net cumulative savings during the fourth year of treatment, and that the net cumulative savings peak after 8 years of galantamine treatment. These benefits are more robust than those reported in the UK, which may reflect regional variations in the acquisition costs of galantamine. For example, in a Swedish analysis, a 19% increase in drug cost would eliminate the predicted savings, whereas in a similar Canadian analysis, the cost would need to be raised by 91% to cancel the net savings.[50]

There is great uncertainty in attempting to compare the available acetylcholinesterase inhibitors by any criteria, particularly those concerning cost. Only preliminary data are available which compare the pharmacoeconomics of galantamine usage with other acetylcholinesterase inhibitors. Nevertheless, these analyses indicate that galantamine use is associated with less time in full-time care and lower treatment costs than are reported for donepezil or rivastigmine.[50,52] Further work in this area may influence future treatment guidelines for Alzheimer's disease, which do not currently make any recommendations regarding the use of one drug over another.[33] Ideally, future pharmacoeconomic evaluations will incorporate measures of the impact on behaviour and activities of daily living into their calculations, as these can have considerable impact over the rate of progression to full-time care. For example, the potential reduction in the consumption of antipsychotics, given the effectiveness of galantamine in reducing non-cognitive symptoms, may add weight to the argument that it is a more economically favourable option than alternative acetylcholinesterase inhibitors.[42]

Preliminary data indicate that galantamine use is associated with less time in full-time care and lower treatment costs than are reported for donepezil or rivastigmine.

Key points

- Galantamine is unique amongst the <u>acetylcholinesterase inhibitors</u> in that it also has a direct effect on <u>nicotinic receptors</u>. Thus, in addition to specifically and reversibly inhibiting acetylcholinesterase, it potentiates the response of nicotinic receptors to <u>acetylcholine</u> and other agonists. These actions serve to reduce the <u>cholinergic</u> deficit associated with Alzheimer's disease.

- Galantamine, at doses of 16, 24 and 32 mg/day, affords benefits over <u>placebo</u> on <u>cognitive</u> function and global improvement.

- Galantamine, at doses of 24 and 32 mg/day, generates improvement in patients' ability to carry out activities of daily living. Data are inconsistent, however, as to the duration of treatment required for this benefit to become significant.

- Data suggest that galantamine improves the behavioural symptoms associated with Alzheimer's disease and also reduces the emergence of new behavioural problems. This may contribute significantly to a reduction in the level of caregiver stress.

- Currently, there are insufficient data from comparative trials to recommend one cholinesterase over another, though the cognitive benefits of galantamine are reported to be more sustained those associated with other acetylcholinesterase inhibitors.

- Further studies are required to determine the relative benefits of individual acetylcholinesterase inhibitors on behavioural and psychological symptoms of Alzheimer's disease.

- The observations relating to galantamine's <u>efficacy</u> made in clinical trials appear to be applicable to naturalistic populations in clinical practice. Benefits of treatment also extend to those patients previously exposed to other acetylcholinesterase inhibitors, to patients with an ApoE 4 <u>genotype</u> and in those with <u>dementia</u> of mixed causes.

- Galantamine is generally well tolerated in the majority of patients. The <u>adverse event</u> profile of galantamine is characteristic of this class of compounds.

- Adverse events are generally mild-to-moderate in severity and gastrointestinal in nature, and occur predominantly during the dose-escalation phase.

- If treatment with galantamine is maintained long-term, the costs of treatment appear to be at least partially offset by the delay in requirement for full-time care.

Any reference made to guidance from the National Institute of Clinical Excellence (NICE) in the preceding section relates to guidelines published in 2001. As we go to press (March 2005), NICE has issued preliminary guidance that is currently under review and will be finalised and published later in 2005 (see Editor's note Pages xx and 127).

References

A list of the published evidence which has been reviewed in compiling the preceding section of *BESTMEDICINE*.

1   Winblad B. Maintaining functional and behavioral abilities in Alzheimer disease. *Alzheimer Dis Assoc Disord* 2001; **15(Suppl 1)**: S34–40.

2   Raskind MA. Update on Alzheimer drugs (galantamine). *Neurologist* 2003; **9**: 235–40.

3   Lanctot KL, Herrmann N, Yau KK *et al.* Efficacy and safety of cholinesterase inhibitors in Alzheimer's disease: a meta-analysis. *Cmaj* 2003; **169**: 557–64.

4   Shigeta M, Homma A. Donepezil for Alzheimer's disease: pharmacodynamic, pharmacokinetic, and clinical profiles. *CNS Drug Rev* 2001; **7**: 353–68.

5   Scott LJ, Goa KL. Galantamine: a review of its use in Alzheimer's disease. *Drugs* 2000; **60**: 1095–122.

6   *Reminyl® (Galantamine). Summary of product characteristics.* Shire Pharmaceuticals Ltd. September, 2004.

7   Samochocki M, Hoffle A, Fehrenbacher A *et al.* Galantamine is an allosterically potentiating ligand of neuronal nicotinic but not of muscarinic acetylcholine receptors. *J Pharmacol Exp Ther* 2003; **305**: 1024–36.

8   Barnes CA, Meltzer J, Houston F *et al.* Chronic treatment of old rats with donepezil or galantamine: effects on memory, hippocampal plasticity and nicotinic receptors. *Neuroscience* 2000; **99**: 17–23.

9   Maelicke A, Albuquerque EX. Allosteric modulation of nicotinic acetylcholine receptors as a treatment strategy for Alzheimer's disease. *Eur J Pharmacol* 2000; **393**: 165–70.

10 Lilienfeld S. Galantamine – a novel cholinergic drug with a unique dual mode of action for the treatment of patients with Alzheimer's disease. *CNS Drug Rev* 2002; **8**: 159–76.

11 Thomsen T, Kewitz H. Selective inhibition of human acetylcholinesterase by galanthamine *in vitro* and *in vivo*. *Life Sci* 1990; **46**: 1553–8.

12 Ritchie CW, Ames D, Clayton T, Lai R. Metaanalysis of randomized trials of the efficacy and safety of donepezil, galantamine, and rivastigmine for the treatment of Alzheimer disease. *Am J Geriatr Psychiatry* 2004; **12**: 358–69.

13 Bickel U, Thomsen T, Weber W *et al.* Pharmacokinetics of galanthamine in humans and corresponding cholinesterase inhibition. *Clin Pharmacol Ther* 1991; **50**: 420–8.

14 Woodruff-Pak DS, Santos IS. Nicotinic modulation in an animal model of a form of associative learning impaired in Alzheimer's disease. *Behav Brain Res* 2000; **113**: 11–19.

15 Sweeney JE, Bachman ES, Coyle JT. Effects of different doses of galanthamine, a long-acting acetylcholinesterase inhibitor, on memory in mice. *Psychopharmacology (Berl)* 1990; **102**: 191–200.

16 Mentis MJ, Sunderland T, Lai J *et al.* Muscarinic versus nicotinic modulation of a visual task. A pet study using drug probes. *Neuropsychopharmacology* 2001; **25**: 555–64.

17 Piotrovsky V, Van Peer A, Van Osselaer N, Armstrong M, Aerssens J. Galantamine population pharmacokinetics in patients with Alzheimer's disease: modeling and simulations. *J Clin Pharmacol* 2003; **43**: 514–23.

18 Jann MW, Shirley KL, Small GW. Clinical pharmacokinetics and pharmacodynamics of cholinesterase inhibitors. *Clin Pharmacokinet* 2002; **41**: 719–39.

19 Mannens GS, Snel CA, Hendrickx J *et al.* The metabolism and excretion of galantamine in rats, dogs, and humans. *Drug Metab Dispos* 2002; **30**: 553–63.

20 Bachus R, Bickel U, Thomsen T, Roots I, Kewitz H. The O-demethylation of the antidementia drug galanthamine is catalysed by cytochrome P450 2D6. *Pharmacogenetics* 1999; **9**: 661–8.

21 Zhao Q, Iyer GR, Verhaeghe T, Truyen L. Pharmacokinetics and safety of galantamine in subjects with hepatic impairment and healthy volunteers. *J Clin Pharmacol* 2002; **42**: 428–36.

22 *British National Formulary (BNF) 48*. London: the British Medical Association and the Royal Pharmaceutical Association of Great Britain. September 2004.

23 Wilkinson D, Murray J. Galantamine: a randomized, double-blind, dose comparison in patients with Alzheimer's disease. *Int J Geriatr Psychiatry* 2001; **16**: 852–7.

24 Wilcock GK, Lilienfeld S, Gaens E. Efficacy and safety of galantamine in patients with mild to moderate Alzheimer's disease: multicentre randomised controlled trial. Galantamine International-1 Study Group. *BMJ* 2000; **321**: 1445–9.

25 Tariot PN, Solomon PR, Morris JC *et al.* A 5-month, randomized, placebo-controlled trial of galantamine in AD. The Galantamine USA-10 Study Group. *Neurology* 2000; **54**: 2269–76.

26 Rockwood K, Mintzer J, Truyen L, Wessel T, Wilkinson D. Effects of a flexible galantamine dose in Alzheimer's disease: a randomised, controlled trial. *J Neurol Neurosurg Psychiatry* 2001; **71**: 589–95.

27 Raskind MA, Peskind ER, Wessel T, Yuan W. Galantamine in AD: A 6-month randomized, placebo-controlled trial with a 6-month extension. The Galantamine USA-1 Study Group. *Neurology* 2000; **54**: 2261–8.

28 Stahl SM, Markowitz JS, Papadopoulos G, Sadik K. Examination of nighttime sleep-related problems during double-blind, placebo-controlled trials of galantamine in patients with Alzheimer's disease. *Curr Med Res Opin* 2004; **20**: 517–24.

29 Cummings JL, Schneider L, Tariot PN, Kershaw PR, Yuan W. Reduction of behavioral disturbances and caregiver distress by galantamine in patients with Alzheimer's disease. *Am J Psychiatry* 2004; **161**: 532–8.

30 Galasko D, Kershaw PR, Schneider L, Zhu Y, Tariot PN. Galantamine maintains ability to perform activities of daily living in patients with Alzheimer's disease. *J Am Geriatr Soc* 2004; **52**: 1070–6.

31 Sano M, Wilcock GK, van Baelen B, Kavanagh S. The effects of galantamine treatment on caregiver time in Alzheimer's disease. *Int J Geriatr Psychiatry* 2003; **18**: 942–50.

32 Marcusson J, Bullock R, Gauthier S, Kurz A, Schwalen S. Galantamine demonstrates efficacy and safety in elderly patients with Alzheimer disease. *Alzheimer Dis Assoc Disord* 2003; **17(Suppl 3)**: S86–91.

33 National Institute for Clinical Excellence. Guidance on the use of donepezil, rivastigmine and galantamine for the treatment of Alzheimer's Disease. 2001. *www.nice.org.uk*

34 Dengiz AN, Kershaw P. The clinical efficacy and safety of galantamine in the treatment of Alzheimer's disease. *CNS Spectr* 2004; **9**: 377–92.

35 Wilcock G, Howe I, Coles H *et al.* A long-term comparison of galantamine and donepezil in the treatment of Alzheimer's disease. *Drugs Aging* 2003; **20**: 777–89.

36 Jones RW, Soininen H, Hager K *et al.* A multinational, randomised, 12-week study comparing the effects of donepezil and galantamine in patients with mild to moderate Alzheimer's disease. *Int J Geriatr Psychiatry* 2004; **19**: 58–67.

37 Raskind MA, Peskind ER, Truyen L, Kershaw P, Damaraju CV. The cognitive benefits of galantamine are sustained for at least 36 months: a long-term extension trial. *Arch Neurol* 2004; **61**: 252–6.

38 Lyketsos CG, Reichman WE, Kershaw P, Zhu Y. Long-term outcomes of galantamine treatment in patients with Alzheimer disease. *Am J Geriatr Psychiatry* 2004; **12**: 473–82.

39 Corey-Bloom J. Galantamine: a review of its use in Alzheimer's disease and vascular dementia. *Int J Clin Pract* 2003; **57**: 219–23.

40 Patterson CE, Passmore AP, Crawford VL. A 6-month open-label study of the effectiveness and tolerability of galantamine in patients with Alzheimer's disease. *Int J Clin Pract* 2004; **58**: 144–8.

41 Joffres C, Bucks RS, Haworth J, Wilcock GK, Rockwood K. Patterns of clinically detectable treatment effects with galantamine: a qualitative analysis. *Dement Geriatr Cogn Disord* 2003; **15**: 26–33.

42 Monsch AU, Giannakopoulos P. Effects of galantamine on behavioural and psychological disturbances and caregiver burden in patients with Alzheimer's disease. *Curr Med Res Opin* 2004; **20**: 931–8.

43 Caramelli P, Chaves ML, Engelhardt E *et al.* Effects of galantamine on attention and memory in Alzheimer's disease measured by computerized neuropsychological tests: results of the Brazilian Multi-Center Galantamine Study (GAL-BRA-01). *Arq Neuropsiquiatr* 2004; **62**: 379–84.

44 Mossello E, Tonon E, Caleri V *et al.* Effectiveness and safety of cholinesterase inhibitors in elderly subjects with Alzheimer's disease: a "real world" study. *Arch Gerontol Geriatr Suppl* 2004: 297–307.

45 Mintzer JE, Kershaw P. The efficacy of galantamine in the treatment of Alzheimer's disease: comparison of patients previously treated with acetylcholinesterase inhibitors to patients with no prior exposure. *Int J Geriatr Psychiatry* 2003; **18**: 292–7.

46 Aerssens J, Raeymaekers P, Lilienfeld S *et al.* APOE genotype: no influence on galantamine treatment efficacy nor on rate of decline in Alzheimer's disease. *Dement Geriatr Cogn Disord* 2001; **12**: 69–77.

47 Kurz AF, Erkinjuntti T, Small GW, Lilienfeld S, Damaraju CR. Long-term safety and cognitive effects of galantamine in the treatment of probable vascular dementia or Alzheimer's disease with cerebrovascular disease. *Eur J Neurol* 2003; **10**: 633–40.

48 Markowitz JS, Gutterman EM, Lilienfeld S, Papadopoulos G. Sleep-related outcomes in persons with mild to moderate Alzheimer disease in a placebo-controlled trial of galantamine. *Sleep* 2003; **26**: 602–6.

49 Ward A, Caro JJ, Getsios D *et al.* Assessment of health economics in Alzheimer's disease (AHEAD): treatment with galantamine in the UK. *Int J Geriatr Psychiatry* 2003; **18**: 740–7.

50 Lyseng-Williamson KA, Plosker GL. Galantamine: a pharmacoeconomic review of its use in Alzheimer's disease. *Pharmacoeconomics* 2002; **20**: 919–42.

51 Caro JJ, Getsios D, Migliaccio-Walle K, Raggio G, Ward A. Assessment of health economics in Alzheimer's disease (AHEAD) based on need for full-time care. *Neurology* 2001; **57**: 964–71.

52 Migliaccio-Walle K, Getsios D, Caro JJ *et al.* Economic evaluation of galantamine in the treatment of mild to moderate Alzheimer's disease in the United States. *Clin Ther* 2003; **25**: 1806–25.

Acknowledgements

Figure 2 is adapted from Lilienfeld, 2002.[10]
Figure 3 is adapted from Wilcock *et al.*, 2000.[24]
Figure 4 is adapted from Wilcock *et al.*, 2003.[35]

4. Drug review – Memantine (Ebixa®)

Dr Eleanor Bull
CSF Medical Communications Ltd

Summary

There is substantial evidence to suggest that the excitatory neurotransmitter, glutamate, plays an important role in learning and memory processes and that over-stimulation of glutamatergic transmission may feature strongly in the neuropathology of Alzheimer's disease. The N-methyl-D-aspartate (NMDA)-receptor antagonist, memantine, was the first drug to be licensed in Europe for the treatment of moderately severe-to-severe Alzheimer's disease. In contrast to other currently available NMDA-receptor blockers, memantine specifically prevents the pathological activation of the NMDA receptor, in this way providing neuroprotection against the toxic effects of glutamatergic over-stimulation, as demonstrated in a number of animal models. In clinical trials in patients with moderately severe-to-severe Alzheimer's disease, memantine has been shown to improve cognition, increase global and functional capabilities and prolong patient independence. However, further longer-term trials are required in order to determine whether memantine actually modifies the progression of Alzheimer's disease. Memantine has a favourable tolerability profile, and the incidence of psychotomimetic side-effects is minimal compared with other drugs of the class (e.g. phencyclidine [PCP] and MK-801).

Introduction

The use of the cholinesterase inhibitors (e.g. donepezil, rivastigmine, galantamine) to restore the cholinergic deficit in patients with mild-to-moderate Alzheimer's dementia is well established. However, treatment with such agents is only effective in about half of the patients for whom it is prescribed, and the available cholinesterase inhibitors are not currently licensed in Europe for the treatment of those patients with more severe presentations of Alzheimer's disease.[1,2] It is estimated that

The excitotoxic damage caused by glutamatergic dysfunction may account, at least in part, for the learning and memory deficits of Alzheimer's disease.

moderate-to-severe Alzheimer's disease accounts for up to 50% of all patients and represents a significant challenge for both physicians and caregivers, since patients are usually entirely dependent on others and show serious functional decline and neuropsychiatric symptoms.[1]

Aside from the cholinergic hypothesis, there is growing evidence that the major excitatory neurotransmitter, glutamate, is also implicated in the pathology of Alzheimer's disease.[3–5] Under normal conditions, glutamate has an important role in synaptic plasticity, long-term potentiation (LTP) and, consequently, learning and memory.[6] However, over-stimulation of glutamatergic neurotransmission has been linked with neurodegeneration – a concept known as excitotoxicity. It has been proposed that the excitotoxic damage caused by glutamatergic dysfunction may account, at least in part, for the learning and memory deficits of Alzheimer's disease.[5,7]

One of the receptors through which glutamate mediates its actions is the NMDA receptor, a ligand-gated ion channel that is permeable to monovalent and divalent cations, including calcium.[8] NMDA-receptor activation results in an influx of calcium ions, which under normal physiological conditions, is integral to the LTP process. However, excessive calcium influx followed by its intracellular accumulation can result in neuronal cell death, which initiates a progressive decline in cognitive function.[8,9] Consequently, NMDA receptors have emerged as potential therapeutic targets for Alzheimer's disease.

Memantine is a voltage-dependent, uncompetitive NMDA-receptor antagonist that appears to selectively inhibit the pathological activation of the NMDA receptor, thus serving a neuroprotective function.[10] Memantine was first investigated in the early 1960s for antidiabetic effects, but no efficacy was shown. Later it was developed for a variety of central nervous system indications (e.g. Parkinson's disease, spasticity), but its NMDA-receptor-blocking action was only discovered in the late 1980s, and is now believed to be its most likely therapeutic action.[11] Since 2002, memantine has been licensed in Europe for the treatment of moderately severe-to-severe Alzheimer's disease.[12] The current review discusses the pharmacological properties of memantine and its efficacy in controlled clinical trials in patients with Alzheimer's disease. Clinical trials of memantine in patients with forms of vascular dementia are beyond the scope of this review and are not discussed here.

☛ *The chemistry of memantine is of essentially academic interest and most healthcare professionals will, like you, skip this section.*

Pharmacology

Chemistry

The chemical structure of memantine (1-amino-3,5-dimethyl-adamantane) is presented in Figure 1. The aminoadamantane family of compounds are chemically atypical owing to their unusual three-dimensional tricyclic structures, and include the antiviral agents amantadine and rimantadine.[13]

Figure 1. The chemical structure of memantine.

1-amino-3, 5-dimethyl-adamantane

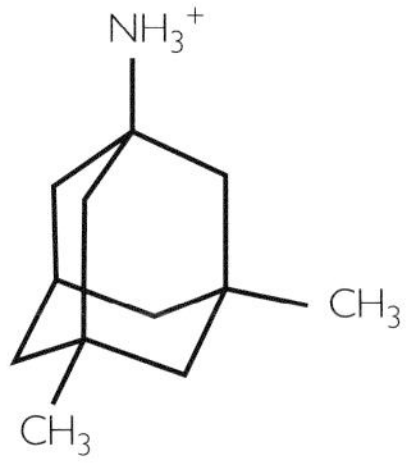

Mechanism of action

Memantine is a voltage-dependent, moderate affinity, uncompetitive NMDA-receptor antagonist.[10] In contrast to other drugs of its class (e.g. PCP and MK-801), memantine appears to selectively block the effects of pathologically elevated tonic levels of glutamate without preventing the physiological activation of the NMDA receptor.[9,10]

Under resting conditions, the NMDA-receptor ion channel is blocked by magnesium ions in a voltage-dependent fashion, such that depolarisation (in the presence of glutamate and glycine [the co-agonist]) is necessary for other ions, including calcium, to pass through the channel.[14] The physiological activation of the NMDA receptor results in the regulated entry of calcium ions, which initiate a number of enzymatic processes that are essential for neuronal memory formation.[8] However, the pathological activation of the receptor, as has been proposed to occur in Alzheimer's disease, results in the accumulation of intracellular calcium, neuronal dysfunction and ultimately cell damage or death. Under these conditions, the 'filtering' capacity of the magnesium ions is not sufficient to prevent the pathological influx of excitotoxic calcium. As depicted in Figure 2, memantine acts as an 'improved magnesium' and blocks the pathological activation of NDMA receptors, acting as a filter to block excessive synaptic noise and thereby restoring synaptic plasticity.[8]

A number of lines of experimental evidence support the role of memantine in improving learning and memory capacity. Thus, memantine:

- restores impairment of synaptic plasticity induced by over-stimulation of NMDA receptors in hippocampal slices at concentrations known to improve cognition in patients with Alzheimer's disease[15]
- attenuates impairment of passive avoidance learning produced by NMDA[15]
- improves learning in rats with lesions of the entorhinal cortex[16]
- prolongs the duration of synaptic plasticity and improves memory retention in the Morris water maze model of spatial memory.[17]

> Memantine acts as an 'improved magnesium' and blocks the pathological activation of NMDA receptors, acting as a filter to block excessive synaptic noise and thereby restoring synaptic plasticity.

Figure 2. Schematic representation of how the fast unblocking kinetics of memantine allow it to differentiate between the physiological and pathological activation of NMDA receptors.[11]

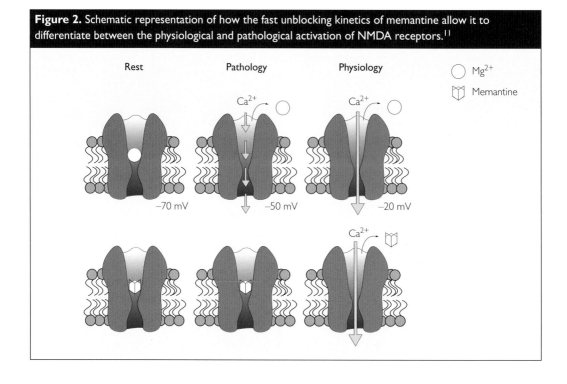

In addition, there is some experimental evidence to show that memantine has neuroprotective properties. Thus, memantine:

- protects against neurodegeneration induced by injection of β-amyloid into the hippocampus in rats[18]
- prevents the deterioration in learning induced by intracerebroventricular infusion of the NMDA-receptor agonist, quinolinic acid[19]
- attenuates the effects of mitochondrial failure induced by injection of the mitochondrial toxin, 3-nitropropionic acid, into the Nucleus Basalis of Meynert (NBM) in rats – a key structure known to be affected in Alzheimer's disease.[20]
- attenuates malonate-induced striatal lesions[21]
- inhibits the abnormal hyperphosphorylation and accumulation of the tau protein in cultured rat hippocampal slices – which forms the basis of the neurofibrillary tangles that characterise the pathology of Alzheimer's disease.[22]

In summary, this evidence indicates that memantine appears to promote synaptic plasticity, whilst also preserving or enhancing memory. In addition, memantine may be neuroprotective against the excitotoxic destruction of cholinergic neurones. Each of these properties occurs with clinically relevant drug concentrations of memantine. Taken together, these data strongly support the potential benefit of memantine in the treatment of neurodegenerative dementia.

Memantine appears to promote synaptic plasticity, whilst also preserving or enhancing memory. In addition, memantine may be neuroprotective against the excitotoxic destruction of cholinergic neurones.

Pharmacokinetics

The pharmacokinetic properties of memantine are summarised in Table 1.[10,23–25] Following oral administration, memantine is completely absorbed from the gastrointestinal tract and exhibits linear pharmacokinetics in the dose range 10–40 mg, although there is significant inter-individual variation in steady-state plasma concentrations.[10,23] Memantine may be administered with or without food and is available both as film-coated tablets and as oral drops for those patients who experience difficulties in swallowing tablets.[10] The recommended starting dose is 5 mg daily during the first week, increased in steps of 5 mg at intervals of 1 week up to a maximum of 10 mg twice daily.[12] Treatment should be initiated and supervised by a physician experienced in the treatment of Alzheimer's disease and a caregiver should be available to regularly monitor drug intake.[10]

Approximately 80% of circulating memantine is in the form of the parent compound.[10] The main metabolites of memantine are N-3,5-dimethyl-gludantan (an isomeric mixture of 4- and 6-hydroxy-memantine) and 1-nitroso-3,5-dimethyl-adamantane. However, neither of these metabolites exhibit NMDA-receptor antagonism. The metabolism of memantine does not involve the cytochrome P450 (CYP) system, as shown by an absence of *in vitro* effects on the CYP1A2, 2A6, 2C9, 2D6, 2E1 or 3A4 isoenzymes.[10] Memantine is eliminated renally and undergoes both renal tubular secretion and re-absorption via cationic transport proteins.[10,23]

Special patient populations

There is significant correlation between the rate of creatinine clearance and the total renal clearance of memantine.[10] Thus, it is recommended

☛ *The pharmacokinetics of a drug are of interest to healthcare professionals because it is important for them to understand the action of a drug on the body over a period of time.*

Table 1. The pharmacokinetic properties of memantine. [10,23–25]

Pharmacokinetic parameter	
Oral bioavailability (%)	100
t_{max} (hours)	3–8
C_{max} (ng/mL)	22–46
Plasma protein binding (%)	45
Volume of distribution (L/kg)	10
CSF/serum ratio	0.52
Steady-state concentration (ng/mL)	70–150
Time to steady-state (days)	11
Total clearance (mL/min/1.73 m^2)	170
$t_{1/2}$ (hours)	60–100
Excretion (%)	99 (urine)

AUC, area under the concentration-time curve; CSF, cerebrospinal fluid; t_{max}, time to reach maximum drug plasma concentration (C_{max}); $t_{1/2}$, elimination half-life.

that for patients with moderate renal impairment, defined as creatinine clearance of 40–60 mL/min/1.73 m^2, the daily dose of memantine should not exceed 10 mg daily.[10] Memantine is not recommended in patients with severe <u>renal</u> impairment (creatinine clearance below 9 mL/min/1.73 m^2), owing to a lack of data in this population.[10]

In addition, the renal elimination rate of memantine may be reduced by a factor of seven to nine under alkaline urine conditions, possibly resulting from significant dietary changes (i.e. switching from a predominantly meat-based diet to a vegetarian diet) or from the massive ingestion of <u>alkalising gastric buffers</u>.[10] Under these circumstances, the careful monitoring of the patient is necessitated. <u>Renal tubulary acidosis (RTA)</u> or severe infections of the urinary tract with *<u>Proteus</u> <u>bacteria</u>* may also affect the elimination of memantine and the careful monitoring of such patients is, therefore, strongly advocated.[10] The <u>pharmacokinetics</u> of memantine have not been studied in patients with significant <u>hepatic</u> impairment and a lack of data preclude its use in children and adolescents.[10] No dosage adjustment is necessary when administering memantine to elderly patients, unless they are renally impaired.[10]

Clinical efficacy

Placebo-controlled studies

The first study to evaluate the efficacy of memantine in patients with moderately severe-to-severe dementia, in a mixed population of patients with dementia, was the 9M-BEST study.[26] The inclusion of patients with Alzheimer's disease and patients with <u>vascular</u> dementia was based on the supposition that in advanced dementia, the symptoms of behaviour and functioning do not differ significantly according to dementia <u>aetiology</u>.[26] The Hachinski Ischaemic Scale (HIS) was used prospectively to distinguish patients with Alzheimer's disease or vascular dementia, with a score of less than five broadly signifying Alzheimer's disease. According to this classification, 79 of the 166 patients (49%) included in the study had Alzheimer's disease and the significance of this, in terms of clinical outcome, was negligible. Patients were eligible for the study if they had a Diagnostic and Statistical Manual of Mental Disorders (DSM-III-R) diagnosis of dementia, were in stages 5–7 of the Global Deterioration Scale (GDS) and had a score lower than ten on the Mini-Mental State Examination (MMSE) scale. Patients received either memantine, 5 mg/day, during the first week, and 10 mg/day thereafter, or <u>placebo</u>, for a 12-week period. The <u>baseline</u> characteristics of the two treatment groups were well matched.

At study endpoint, the primary <u>efficacy</u> criterion – the Clinical Global Impression of Change (CGI-C) – showed a clear treatment difference that favoured memantine. The percentage of patients rated as showing 'minimal improvement' (score 3) on the CGI-C were 52 and 35%, for memantine and placebo, respectively, and the percentage of those patients considered 'much improved' (score 2) were 21 *vs* 11%, respectively. The difference in responders 73 *vs* 45% was highly significant in favour of memantine (*p*<0.001). Caregiver dependence, rated using a subscore of the Behavioural Rating Scale for Geriatric Patients (BGP), improved by 3.1 points following memantine treatment and by 1.1 points in those receiving <u>placebo</u> (*p*=0.016 for memantine *vs* placebo). When patients were stratified according to HIS score (i.e. Alzheimer's disease or vascular dementia), no significant differences were reported between low and high HIS scores, either in terms of the CGI-C response rate (73 *vs* 73% of memantine- and 42 *vs* 48% of placebo-treated patients were responders, for HIS<5 and HIS≥5 subgroups, respectively) or the BGP care-dependence subscore. Patients' response to treatment, as measured by the D-scale – a descriptive rating of behavioural activities and functioning in demented geriatric patients – is illustrated in Figure 3. The <u>adverse event</u> rate was similar between treatment groups, with 22% of memantine- and 21% of placebo-treated patients reporting adverse events.

A 28-week <u>double-blind</u> study conducted in the US, examined the therapeutic benefit of memantine in 252 patients with moderate-to-severe Alzheimer's disease, defined according to DSM-IV criteria.[27] Eligibility for recruitment into the study was dependent on an MMSE

> The CGI-C showed a clear treatment difference that favoured memantine.

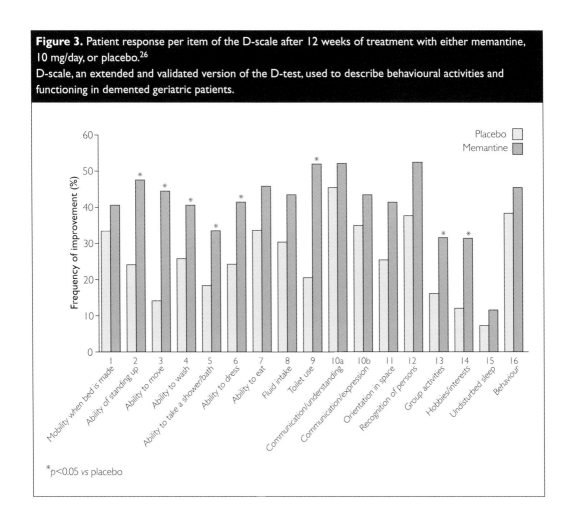

Figure 3. Patient response per item of the D-scale after 12 weeks of treatment with either memantine, 10 mg/day, or placebo.[26]
D-scale, an extended and validated version of the D-test, used to describe behavioural activities and functioning in demented geriatric patients.

*p<0.05 *vs* placebo

score of 3–14, a stage 5 or 6 on the GDS and a stage 6a or greater on the Functional Assessment Staging Instrument. At baseline, the mean MMSE score was 7.9 and the mean patient age was 76 years. Patients received memantine, 20 mg/day, or placebo, for a period of 28 weeks. Of the 252 patients initially enrolled in the study, 71 terminated treatment prematurely (23 vs 33% patients, for memantine and placebo, respectively). The changes in Clinician's Interview-Based Impression of Change Plus Caregiver Input (CIBIC-Plus) and Alzheimer's Disease Cooperative Study Activities of Daily Living Inventory (ADCS-ADLsev) are shown in Figure 4. Overall, clinical outcome was significantly better than placebo following memantine treatment (CIBIC-Plus, p=0.03; ADCS-ADLsev, p=0.003 for observed-cases [OC] analyses). The Severe Impairment Battery (SIB) also highlighted significant improvements in patients' outcomes following memantine treatment compared with placebo (change from baseline: –4 vs –10 for memantine and placebo, respectively; p<0.001, last observation carried forward [LOCF]). In addition, the percentage of patients responding to treatment – defined as the proportion who improved or showed no deterioration on the CIBIC-Plus, ADCS-ADLsev and/or SIB – measured 29 vs 10%, for memantine and placebo, respectively (p=0.0004). The frequency of adverse events was comparable between treatment groups, with 84% of memantine- and 87% of placebo-treated patients reporting adverse events. More patients receiving placebo than patients receiving memantine discontinued treatment prematurely as a result of adverse events (17 vs 10%, respectively; p-value not reported).

These placebo-controlled studies have formed the basis for further analyses, which have highlighted improvements in functional ability and patient independence following treatment with memantine.[28,29]

In one such investigation, patients from the study by Reisberg et al. described previously (n=252),[27] were classified according to their ADCS-ADLsev ratings and further subdivided on the basis of their basic and instrumental ADL capabilities (B-ADL and I-ADL).[27,28] B-ADL scores were calculated as the sum of all basic activities (e.g. eating, walking, bathing, grooming, dressing and toileting) whilst I-ADL scores described more complex activities (e.g. using the telephone, preparing a meal, doing the washing). These scores were used to determine the independence of the patient after 28 weeks of treatment with either memantine or placebo. Overall, dependent patients (42% of the study population) showed longer disease duration, poorer cognition, greater disease severity, more behavioural alterations, and higher societal costs than independent patients (58% of the study population). After controlling for autonomy and disease severity at baseline, memantine-treated patients were three-times more likely than placebo-treated patients to remain independent after 28 weeks of treatment. These data provide evidence that memantine enhances independence in patients with moderate-to-severe Alzheimer's disease and delays the patient's transition to the stage of the disease when they are likely to become dependent on a caregiver.

The percentage of patients responding to treatment measured 29 vs 10%, for memantine and placebo, respectively (p<0.001).

Memantine-treated patients were three-times more likely than placebo-treated patients to remain independent after 28 weeks of treatment.

Figure 4. Change from baseline in the Clinician's Interview-Based Impression of Change Plus Caregiver Input (CIBIC-Plus) global scores (top) and in the Alzheimer's Disease Cooperative Study Activities of Daily Living Inventory, modified for severe dementia (ADCS-ADLsev; bottom).[27]

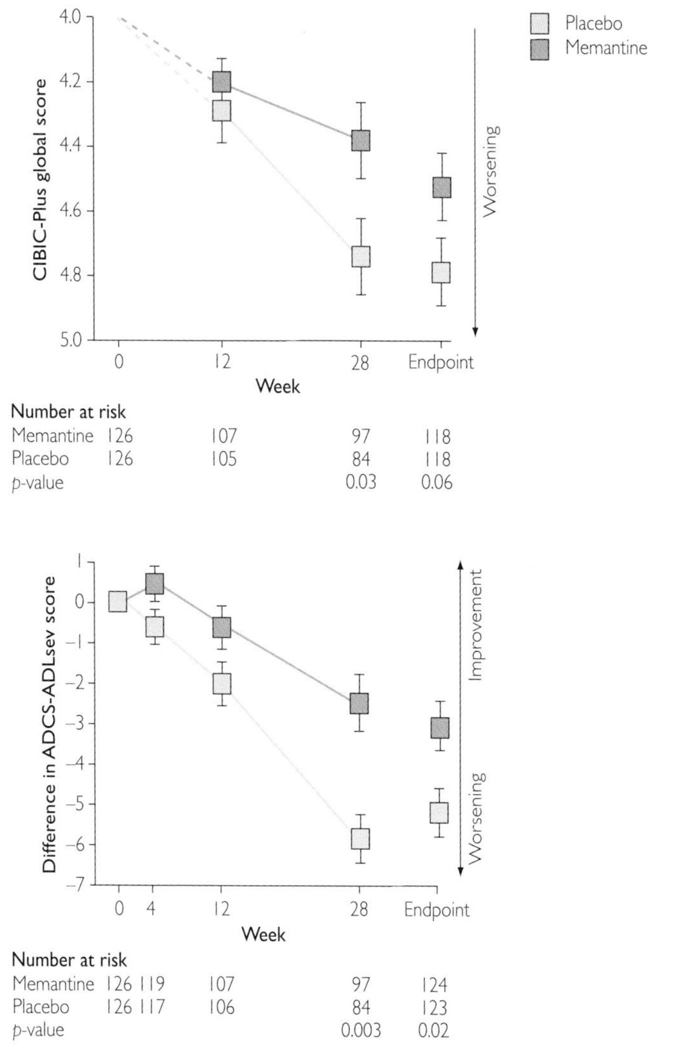

Number at risk

Memantine	126	107	97	118
Placebo	126	105	84	118
p-value			0.03	0.06

Number at risk

Memantine	126	119	107	97	124
Placebo	126	117	106	84	123
p-value				0.003	0.02

Safety and tolerability

In general, memantine is well tolerated amongst patients with Alzheimer's disease and adverse events are usually mild-to-moderate in severity.[10] Reported side-effects of memantine treatment have included dizziness, diarrhoea, insomnia, confusion, headache, hallucinations and tiredness. Less frequently reported adverse events have included

You are strongly urged to consult your doctor before taking, stopping or changing any of the products reviewed or referred to in *BESTMEDICINE* or any other medication that has been prescribed or recommended by your doctor.

vomiting, anxiety, increased muscle tone, cystitis and increased libido.[10,12,23] Table 2 presents the adverse events most frequently reported in controlled clinical trials of memantine.[10]

In contrast with some other NMDA-receptor antagonists (e.g. PCP, MK-801), memantine is associated with minimal psychotomimetic side-effects (e.g. delusions, hallucinations and depersonalisation), ataxia and motor incoordination, providing that the dose is properly titrated over a period of 3–4 weeks.[11] The fast unblocking kinetics of memantine described previously are likely to account for its improved tolerability over other drugs in this class.[30,31]

Drug interactions

As discussed previously, memantine is associated with minimal inhibition of CYP enzymes and thus undergoes limited interaction with drugs that inhibit the CYP system.[31] However, the risk of pharmacotoxic psychosis prohibits the concomitant use of memantine with other NMDA-receptor antagonists (e.g. amantadine, ketamine and dextromethorphan).[10,12]

Potential and/or confirmed drug interactions associated with memantine that also merit consideration when prescribing the drug include:
- enhanced effects of L-dopa, dopaminergic agonists and anticholinergics
- reduced effects of barbiturates and neuroleptics

> The risk of pharmacotoxic psychosis prohibits the concomitant use of memantine with other NMDA-receptor antagonists (e.g. amantadine, ketamine and dextromethorphan).

Table 2. The most frequently observed adverse events associated with memantine (>4% for memantine) in patients with moderately severe-to-severe Alzheimer's disease.[10]

Adverse event	Incidence of adverse event (%)	
	Placebo (n=288)	Memantine (n=299)
Agitation	17.4	9.0
Inflicted injury	6.9	6.7
Urinary incontinence	7.3	5.7
Diarrhoea	4.9	5.4
Insomnia	4.9	5.4
Dizziness	2.8	5.0
Headache	3.1	5.0
Hallucination	2.1	5.0
Fall	4.9	4.7
Constipation	4.5	4.0
Coughing	5.9	4.0

- modified effects of <u>antispasmodic agents</u> (e.g. dantrolene, baclofen)
- modified effects of drugs that use the same <u>renal</u> cationic transport system as amantadine (e.g. cimetidine, ranitidine, procainamide, quinidine, quinine, nicotine)
- reduced serum levels of the thiazide diuretic, hydrochlorothiazide.[10]

Contra-indications

In view of its pharmacological profile, memantine should be administered with caution to patients with epilepsy.[10] Although it is unlikely that patients with advanced Alzheimer's disease would be regularly performing skilled tasks, driving or operating heavy machinery, they should be advised of the changes in reactivity associated with memantine treatment.[10] A lack of data limits the use of memantine in patients having undergone recent <u>myocardial infarction</u>, or those with uncompensated congestive heart failure or uncontrolled <u>hypertension</u>.[10]

Pharmacoeconomics

Patients in the advanced stages of Alzheimer's disease are increasingly dependent on others for all aspects of their day-to-day functioning. Consequently, the financial and emotional demands on patients and their caregivers and the costs imposed on nursing homes are immense. Compared with the economic implications of the number of days spent in nursing homes or hospitals, the hours of home support and the burden of informal care, the cost of antidementia medication is relatively minor.

The 28-week clinical efficacy trial by Reisberg *et al.* in 252 patients with moderate-to-severe Alzheimer's disease, also incorporated a resource utilisation and cost analysis.[27,32] Overall, patients treated with memantine required significantly less caregiver time than those receiving <u>placebo</u>, a difference amounting to 51.5 hours per month ($p=0.02$ *vs* placebo).[32] Memantine also prolonged the transition to institutionalisation, as demonstrated by the transfer of only one memantine-treated patient into an institutional setting during the course of the study, compared with five <u>placebo</u>-treated patients ($p=0.04$). Total costs to society were also significantly lower in the memantine-treatment group (a difference of US$1090 per month; $p=0.01$ *vs* placebo). The main reasons for this difference were derived from reductions in total caregiver costs and direct non-medical costs. As expected, the direct medical costs were significantly higher in the memantine treatment group compared with placebo ($p<0.01$).

The effect of treatment with memantine on resource utilisation and total healthcare costs over a 2-year period was investigated using a <u>Markov model</u>, with transition probabilities derived from the 28-week clinical <u>efficacy</u> trial by Reisberg *et al.*[27,33] Compared with no treatment, memantine was associated with greater cost-effectiveness, in terms of

> Patients treated with memantine required significantly less caregiver time than those receiving placebo, a difference amounting to 51.5 hours per month.

patient independence, years spent in the community and quality
adjusted life-years (QALYs). The most significant benefit was observed
in those patients with an MMSE score of greater than 10 who were
maintaining their independence.

Key points

- Memantine is a <u>voltage-dependent</u>, uncompetitive NMDA-receptor antagonist indicated for the treatment of patients with moderately severe-to-severe Alzheimer's disease.

- The potential benefit of NMDA-receptor antagonists such as memantine in Alzheimer's disease follows the strong association between pathological over-stimulation of glutamatergic neurotransmission and excitotoxic neurodegeneration.

- In contrast to other drugs of its class (e.g. PCP and MK-801), memantine selectively targets the pathologically activated NMDA receptor, thus preventing the cellular influx of potentially excitotoxic <u>calcium ions</u> without disrupting physiological receptor functioning.

- Memantine demonstrates linear <u>pharmacokinetics</u> over its recommended dose range and is associated with minimal drug–<u>drug interactions</u>.

- In clinical trials, memantine elicited significant improvements and/or stabilisation in global measures of clinical change and slowed the rate of deterioration of patients with advanced Alzheimer's disease compared with <u>placebo</u>.

- The SIB, as a measure of cognition, revealed significant patient benefit over placebo after 28 weeks of memantine administration.

- The ability with which patients performed daily tasks was significantly improved and/or stabilised by memantine over treatment periods of 12 and 28 weeks. There is also evidence that shows patients maintain their independence for longer following memantine treatment.

- Memantine is not associated with a high frequency of psychotomimetic side-effects, in contrast to other drugs of its class, perhaps as a consequence of its fast NMDA-receptor-blocking/-unblocking <u>kinetics</u>.

Any reference made to guidance from the National Institute of Clinical Excellence (NICE) in the preceding section relates to guidelines published in 2001. As we go to press (March 2005), NICE has issued preliminary guidance that is currently under review and will be finalised and published later in 2005 (see Editor's note Pages xx and 127).

References

A list of the published evidence which has been reviewed in compiling the preceding section of *BESTMEDICINE*.

1   Voisin T, Reynish E, Portet F, Feldman H, Vellas B. What are the treatment options for patients with severe Alzheimer's disease? *CNS Drugs* 2004; **18**: 575–83.

2   Wilcock G. Memantine for the treatment of dementia. *Lancet Neurol* 2003; **2**: 503–5.

3   Palmer A, Gershon S. Is the neuronal basis of Alzheimer's disease cholinergic or glutamatergic? *FASEB J* 1990; **4**: 2745–52.

4   Muller W, Mutschler E, Riederer P. Noncompetitive NMDA receptor antagonists with fast open-channel blocking kinetics and strong voltage-dependency as potential therapeutic agents for Alzheimer's dementia. *Pharmacopsychiatry* 1995; **28**: 113–24.

5   Greenamyre J, Maragos W, Albin R, Penney J, Young A. Glutamate transmission and toxicity in Alzheimer's disease. *Prog Neuropsychopharmacol Biol Psychiatry* 1988; **12**: 421–30.

6   Bliss T, Collingridge G. A synaptic model of memory: long-term potentiation in the hippocampus. *Nature* 1993; **361**: 31–9.

7   Danysz W, Parsons C, Mobius H, Stoffler A, Quack G. Neuroprotective and symptomatological action of memantine relevant for Alzheimer's disease – a unified hypothesis on the mechanism of action. *Neurotox Res* 2000; **2**: 85–98.

8   Danysz W, Parsons C. The NMDA receptor antagonist memantine as a symptomatological and neuroprotective treatment for Alzheimer's disease: preclinical evidence. *Int J Geriatr Psychiatry* 2003; **18**: S23–32.

9   Scarpini E, Scheltens P, Feldman H. Treatment of Alzheimer's disease: current status and new perspectives. *Lancet Neurol* 2003; **2**: 539–47.

10 *Ebixa® (Memantine). Summary of product characteristics.* Lundbeck Ltd. 2003.

11 Parsons C, Danysz W, Quack G. Memantine is a clinically well tolerated N-methyl-D-aspartate (NMDA) receptor antagonist – a review of preclinical data. *Neuropharmacology* 1999; **38**: 735–67.

12 *British National Formulary (BNF) 48.* London: British Medical Association and Royal Pharmaceutical Society of Great Britain, September, 2004.

13 Rogawski M, Wenk G. The neuropharmacological basis for the use of memantine in the treatment of Alzheimer's disease. *CNS Drug Rev* 2003; **9**: 275–308.

14 Mayer M, Westbrook G, Guthrie P. Voltage-dependent block by Mg2+ of NMDA responses in spinal cord neurones. *Nature* 1984; **309**: 261–3.

15 Zajaczkowski W, Frankiewicz T, Parsons C, Danysz W. Uncompetitive NMDA receptor antagonists attenuate NMDA-induced impairment of passive avoidance learning and LTP. *Neuropharmacology* 1997; **36**: 961–71.

16 Zajaczkowski W, Quack G, Danysz W. Infusion of (+) - MK-801 and memantine – contrasting effects on radial maze learning in rats with entorhinal cortex lesion. *Eur J Pharmacol* 1996; **296**: 239–46.

17 Barnes C, Danysz W, Parsons C. Effects of the uncompetitive NMDA receptor antagonist memantine on hippocampal long-term potentiation, short-term exploratory modulation and spatial memory in awake, freely moving rats. *Eur J Neurosci* 1996; **8**: 565–71.

18 Miguel-Hidalgo J, Alvarez X, Cacabelos R, Quack G. Neuroprotection by memantine against neurodegeneration induced by beta-amyloid(1-40). *Brain Res* 2002; **958**: 210–21.

19 Misztal M, Frankiewicz T, Parsons C, Danysz W. Learning deficits induced by chronic intraventricular infusion of quinolinic acid – protection by MK-801 and memantine. *Eur J Pharmacol* 1996; **296**: 1–8.

20 Wenk G, Danysz W, Roice D. The effects of mitochondrial failure upon cholinergic toxicity in the nucleus basalis. *Neuroreport* 1996; **7**: 1453–6.

21 Schulz J, Matthews R, Henshaw D, Beal M. Neuroprotective strategies for treatment of lesions produced by mitochondrial toxins: implications for neurodegenerative diseases. *Neuroscience* 1996; **71**: 1043–8.

22 Li L, Sengupta A, Haque N, Grundke-Iqbal I, Iqbal K. Memantine inhibits and reverses the Alzheimer type abnormal hyperphosphorylation of tau and associated neurodegeneration. *FEBS Lett* 2004; **566**: 261–9.

23 Jarvis B, Figgitt D. Memantine. *Drugs Aging* 2003; **20**: 465–76.

24 Kornhuber J, Quack G. Cerebrospinal fluid and serum concentrations of the N-methyl-D-aspartate (NMDA) receptor antagonist memantine in man. *Neurosci Lett* 1995; **195**: 137–9.

25 Prasher V. Review of donepezil, rivastigmine, galantamine and memantine for the treatment of dementia in Alzheimer's disease in adults with Down syndrome: implications for the intellectual disability population. *Int J Geriatr Psychiatry* 2004; **19**: 509–15.

26 Winblad B, Poritis N. Memantine in severe dementia: results of the 9M-Best Study (Benefit and efficacy in severely demented patients during treatment with memantine). *Int J Geriatr Psychiatry* 1999; **14**: 135–46.

27 Reisberg B, Doody R, Stoffler A *et al.* Memantine in moderate-to-severe Alzheimer's disease. *N Engl J Med* 2003; **348**: 1333–41.

28 Rive B, Vercelletto M, Damier F, Cochran J, Francois C. Memantine enhances autonomy in moderate to severe Alzheimer's disease. *Int J Geriatr Psychiatry* 2004; **19**: 458–64.

29 Doody R, Wirth Y, Schmitt F, Mobius H. Specific functional effects of memantine treatment in patients with moderate to severe Alzheimer's disease. *Dement Geriatr Cogn Disord* 2004; **18**: 227–32.

30 Kornhuber J, Weller M. Psychotogenicity and N-methyl-D-aspartate receptor antagonism: implications for neuroprotective pharmacotherapy. *Biol Psychiatry.* 1997; **41**: 135–44.

31 Doraiswamy P. Alzheimer's disease and the glutamate NMDA receptor. *Psychopharmacol Bull* 2003; **37**: 41–9.

32 Wimo A, Winblad B, Stoffler A, Wirth Y, Mobius H. Resource utilisation and cost analysis of memantine in patients with moderate to severe Alzheimer's disease. *Pharmacoeconomics* 2003; **21**: 327–40.

33 Jones R, McCrone P, Guilhaume C. Cost effectiveness of memantine in Alzheimer's disease : an analysis based on a probabilistic Markov model from a UK perspective. *Drugs Aging* 2004; **21**: 607–20.

Acknowledgements

Figure 2 is adapted from Parsons *et al.,* 1999.[11]
Figure 3 is adapted from Winblad *et al.,* 1999.[26]
Figure 4 is adapted from Reisberg *et al.,* 2003.[27]

5. Drug review – Rivastigmine (Exelon®)

Dr Eleanor Bull
CSF Medical Communications Ltd

Summary

Rivastigmine is a <u>pseudo-irreversible</u> <u>cholinesterase inhibitor</u> indicated for the symptomatic treatment of patients with mild-to-moderate Alzheimer's disease. By inhibiting the enzymatic degradation of <u>acetylcholine</u> by acetyl- and <u>butyrylcholinesterase</u>, rivastigmine partially restores the deficit in <u>cholinergic</u> activity that characterises Alzheimer's disease, and thereby improves or stabilises cognition and also improves day-to-day functioning of patients with the disorder. Rivastigmine exerts its pharmacological effects selectively on the central nervous system, and preferentially on the <u>monomeric G1</u> <u>isoform</u> of <u>acetylcholinesterase</u> that is more abundant in the brains of patients with Alzheimer's disease. The duration of action of rivastigmine persists for much longer than the drug resides in the plasma, owing to its slow dissociation from the <u>esteratic</u> site of cholinesterase – a so-called pseudo-irreversible <u>mechanism of action</u>. In <u>placebo-controlled</u> clinical trials, rivastigmine has been shown to have a significant benefit on the three key areas most affected in Alzheimer's disease; cognition, global functioning and activities of daily living (ADL). In addition rivastigmine may also alleviate non-<u>cognitive</u> symptoms of Alzheimer's disease such as delusions and perceptual disturbance. <u>Open-label</u> extensions of published clinical trials have provided preliminary evidence of continuing clinical benefit with rivastigmine. Early intervention with rivastigmine has also been shown to be favourable from an economic perspective. To date, placebo-controlled trials that explore the efficacy of rivastigmine beyond 6 months, head-to-head comparative trials and studies that examine its effects on disease progression, have not yet reported. Rivastigmine is generally well tolerated with the majority of treatment-related <u>adverse events</u> being gastrointestinal in nature (e.g. nausea, vomiting, diarrhoea) and mild-to-moderate in severity.

Introduction

The most prominent feature of Alzheimer's disease is the loss of cholinergic neurones and therapeutic strategies have focused on cholinergic activation. The cholinergic hypothesis of Alzheimer's disease links the deficit in central cholinergic transmission, caused by the degeneration of basal forebrain nuclei, with the cognitive, global and behavioural decline that characterise the disease.[1]

Potentially, a number of different strategies would restore cholinergic function and thus offer symptomatic benefits to patients with Alzheimer's disease. In the past, however, drugs which increased acetylcholine synthesis, augmented presynaptic acetylcholine release or stimulated postsynaptic muscarinic and nicotinic receptors failed to demonstrate any therapeutic benefit.[2] By far the most successful pharmacological agents to date have been the cholinesterase inhibitors (e.g. donepezil, galantamine, rivastigmine and tacrine[a]), which inhibit the enzymatic degradation of acetylcholine in the synaptic cleft. Cholinesterase inhibition aims to maximise the effectiveness of the remaining cholinergic neurotransmission by preventing enzymatic hydrolysis of the reduced amounts of neurotransmitter that are released.

Currently, the cholinesterase inhibitors represent the standard treatment option for mild-to-moderate Alzheimer's disease and have been shown to improve cognition, behavioural symptoms and global functioning of patients with the disorder.[1] The only other drug to be licensed for Alzheimer's disease is memantine, a NMDA-receptor antagonist used for the treatment of patients with moderate-to-severe disease.

The widespread use of the first-generation cholinesterase inhibitors (e.g. physostigmine and tacrine) has been hampered as a consequence of their detrimental effects on hepatic and cardiovascular function in conjunction with a high propensity for drug–drug interactions. This meant that dosage regimens of these agents may have been suboptimal to the detriment of significant therapeutic benefit.[3] The second-generation compounds (e.g. donepezil, galantamine and rivastigmine) have demonstrated improved tolerability and safety.

Rivastigmine was first licensed in the UK in 1998 and is indicated for the symptomatic treatment of mild-to-moderately severe Alzheimer's disease.[4] Rivastigmine facilitates cholinergic neurotransmission by slowing the degradation of acetylcholine catalysed by the acetyl- and butyrylcholinesterase enzymes. The relatively slow dissociation of rivastigmine from the esteratic site of the enzyme prolongs its pharmacological effects. As such, this mechanism of action is described as pseudo-irreversible.[4]

According to current guidelines, treatment with rivastigmine should be initiated and supervised by a physician experienced in the diagnosis and treatment of Alzheimer's disease.[4] Patients should be maintained on their maximum tolerated dose within the therapeutic dose range (up to a total of 12 mg/day, administered in two daily doses) for as long as a

> The cholinesterase inhibitors represent the standard treatment option for mild-to-moderate Alzheimer's disease and have been shown to improve cognition, behavioural symptoms and global functioning.

> Rivastigmine facilitates cholinergic neurotransmission by slowing the degradation of acetylcholine catalysed by the acetyl- and butyrylcholinesterase enzymes.

---

[a]Tacrine is not currently licensed in the UK.

clinical benefit is observed, with regular re-assessment.[4,5] The current review discusses the pharmacological properties of rivastigmine and its efficacy in controlled clinical trials in patients with mild-to-moderate Alzheimer's disease. Clinical trials of rivastigmine in patients with vascular dementia are beyond the scope of the review and are not discussed herein.

Pharmacology

Chemistry

The chemical structure of rivastigmine – a carbamate derivative – is illustrated in Figure 1.

Mechanism of action

Rivastigmine is an inhibitor of both acetyl- and butyrylcholinesterase enzymes in the central nervous system (CNS) and demonstrates limited peripheral activity.[4,6] Through inhibition of these enzymes and consequent limitation of the degradation of acetylcholine, rivastigmine increases available acetylcholine and enhances cholinergic function in intact neurones, thereby reversing the pathological cholinergic deficit in Alzheimer's disease.

The inhibition of butyrylcholinesterase is unique to rivastigmine since donepezil and galantamine only inhibit acetylcholinesterase. Both acetyl- and butyrylcholinesterase are involved in the enzymatic degradation of acetylcholine in the CNS. In normal human brain, butyrylcholinesterase constitutes 10% of total cholinesterase activity and is mainly associated with glial cells.[7] As Alzheimer's disease progresses, cortical neurones are lost and acetylcholinesterase activity decreases by up to 45%, whilst the activity of butyrylcholinesterase in certain brain areas (e.g. the cerebral cortex) increases by 40–90%.[8,9] Although the role of buytyrylcholinesterase inhibition has yet to be fully elucidated, the dual enzyme inhibition by rivastigmine may ultimately result in more pronounced cholinesterase inhibition in the brain than that offered by acetylcholinesterase-specific drugs (e.g. donepezil).[1]

The inhibition of cholinesterases by rivastigmine is 'pseudo-irreversible', that is to say, the duration of the effect persists for much

☛ The chemistry of rivastigmine is of essentially academic interest and most healthcare professionals will, like you, skip this section.

Figure 1. The chemical structure of rivastigmine.

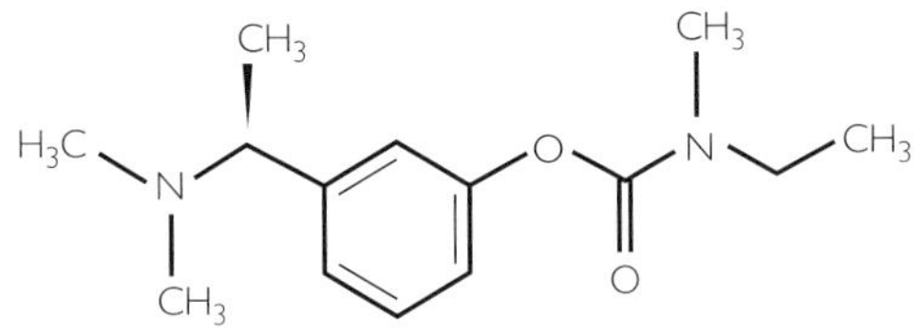

longer than the drug resides in the plasma.[6] Rivastigmine binds to the esteratic site of the cholinesterase enzymes which undergoes carbamylation, thus forming a covalently bound complex that temporarily inactivates the enzyme.[4] The carbamyl moiety of rivastigmine remains bound for much longer than the acetyl moiety of the endogenous ligand, acetylcholine, and this delays the regeneration of the active enzyme.[6]

The major form of acetylcholinesterase in the hippocampal and cortical regions of the brain is G4 – a globular, tetrameric enzyme. Under normal physiological conditions, the monomeric G1 isoform is less abundant, although in patients with Alzheimer's disease, G4 is selectively lost and the G1 isoform predominates.[2,6] Rivastigmine preferentially inhibits the G1 variant of acetylcholinesterase and so its inhibitory effects increase as Alzheimer's disease progresses.[10]

> Rivastigmine preferentially inhibits the G1 variant of acetylcholinesterase and so its inhibitory effects increase as Alzheimer's disease progresses.

Cognitive effects of cholinesterase inhibition

The relationship between the cognitive effects of rivastigmine, 1–6 mg/day, and its inhibition of acetyl- and butyrylcholinesterase in cerebrospinal fluid (CSF), was examined in 18 patients with mild-to-moderate Alzheimer's disease.[11] Significant correlation was detected between the change in Computerised Neuropsychological Test Battery (CNTB) summary scores, used as measure of cognitive function, and the inhibition of both acetyl- and butyrylcholinesterase (r=–0.56 and r=–0.65, respectively; $p<0.05$ and $p<0.01$). Interestingly, improvements in speed, attention and memory-related subtests of the CNTB correlated significantly with the degree of inhibition of butyrylcholinesterase but not acetylcholinesterase in the CSF (choice reaction time 0.403 and 0.501 for acetyl- and butyrylcholinesterase respectively, $p<0.05$ for butyrylcholinesterase only; delayed recall, –0.36 and –0.69, respectively, $p<0.01$ for butyrylcholinesterase only; visual memory –0.42 vs –0.52, respectively, $p<0.05$ for butyrylcholinesterase only).

A similar study examined the relationship between neuropsychological symptoms and plasma cholinesterase activity in 11 patients with mild Alzheimer's disease receiving rivastigmine, 3–12 mg/day, compared with 21 untreated patients with Alzheimer's disease and 22 patients with mild cognitive impairment, over a period of 12 months.[12] At the end of the study, cognitive function had declined slightly in Alzheimer's disease patients treated with rivastigmine, yet worsened markedly in untreated patients (mean change in Mini Mental State Examination [MMSE] score from baseline –1.2 *vs* –3.4 for treated and untreated patients, respectively; $p=0.01$). There was a positive and significant correlation between mean z-scores of cognitive function and plasma cholinesterase inhibition amongst rivastigmine-treated patients after 3 and 6 months of treatment (r=0.64 and r=0.61 for 3 and 6 months, respectively; $p=0.03$ and $p=0.05$).

> There was a positive and significant correlation between mean z-scores of cognitive function and plasma cholinesterase inhibition amongst rivastigmine-treated patients.

Brain metabolic effects

Brain imaging of patients with mild-to-moderate Alzheimer's disease has revealed significant changes in cerebral blood flow and brain metabolism associated with rivastigmine treatment.

- Rivastigmine-treated patients (n=27) who showed improvement or stabilisation on the Clinical Interview Based Impression of Change plus Caregiver Input (CIBIC-plus) scale after 26 weeks, also showed a marked increase in brain metabolism involving, in part, memory-related cortices and the prefrontal system ($p<0.01$), as determined by positron emission tomography using [^{18}F]-flurodeoxyglucose (FDG-PET).[13]
- Cerebral glucose metabolism increased significantly over 12 months in rivastigmine-treated patients (n=11) compared with those patients receiving tacrine or no treatment (n=38).[14]
- Regional cerebral blood flow increased in rivastigmine-treated patients (n=25) but decreased in untreated patients (n=8) over a 12-month period, as determined by Single Photon Emission Computed Tomography (SPECT).[15]

Pharmacokinetics

The pharmacokinetic properties of rivastigmine are presented in Table 1.[2,4,6] Rivastigmine crosses the blood–brain barrier and is quickly detected in CSF following oral twice-daily administration. Consistent with its non-linear pharmacokinetic profile, rivastigmine exhibits increased bioavailability with increased dose in patients with mild-to-moderate Alzheimer's disease.[16]

The marked difference between the pharmacokinetic and pharmacodynamic half-lives of rivastigmine (1–2 *vs* 10 hours,

☛ *The pharmacokinetics of a drug are of interest to healthcare professionals because it is important for them to understand the action of a drug on the body over a period of time.*

Table 1. The pharmacokinetic properties of rivastigmine.[2,4,6]	
Pharmacokinetic parameter	
Oral bioavailability (%)	36
t_{max} (hours)	0.8–1.2
C_{max} (µg/L)	↓ by 30% by food
AUC (µg/L.hour)	↑ by 30% by food
Volume of distribution (L/kg)	1.8–2.7
Plasma-protein binding (%)	~40
$t_{1/2}$ (hours)	1–2 (pharmacokinetic)
	10 (pharmacodynamic)
Total plasma clearance (L/hour)	70 (after a 2.7 mg i.v. dose)
Excretion (%)	>90 (urine)
	<1 (faeces)

AUC, area under the concentration-time curve; i.v., intravenous; t_{max}, time to reach maximum drug plasma concentration (C_{max}); $t_{1/2}$, elimination half-life.

respectively) is attributable to its <u>pseudo-irreversible</u> <u>mechanism of action</u>. Rivastigmine dissociates from the <u>esteratic</u> site of the <u>acetylcholinesterase</u> <u>enzyme</u> more slowly than <u>acetylcholine</u>, and therefore, its inhibitory effects are prolonged for longer than the short plasma half-life would predict.[2] This allows for a twice-daily dosing schedule.

The effective dose of rivastigmine ranges between 3 and 6 mg administered on a twice-daily basis. Dosing with rivastigmine should be initiated at a dose of 1.5 mg twice daily and then gradually increased according to the individual patient's response and tolerability, in 1.5 mg increments, up to a maximum of 6 mg twice daily, at minimum intervals of 2 weeks. Recent experience in clinical practice suggests that a 4-week <u>titration</u> interval may further minimise gastrointestinal <u>adverse events</u>. If the dosage regimen is interrupted for a period of several days, treatment should be re-started at 1.5 mg twice daily and re-titrated as previously.[4,17] Although some effect of food on the pharmacokinetics of rivastigmine is evident from the delay in the time (t_{max}) to reach maximum drug plasma concentration (C_{max}), rivastigmine should be administered with morning and evening meals.[4]

Metabolism

Rivastigmine is rapidly and extensively <u>metabolised</u>, primarily by cholinesterase-mediated hydrolysis, to the decarbamylated inactive metabolite, NAP 226–90.[2,4] NAP 226-90 is metabolised through the liver by <u>N-demethylation</u> or <u>sulphate conjugation</u> and excreted through the kidneys. Since the metabolism of rivastigmine occurs primarily at the <u>synapse</u> rather than in the liver, the major <u>cytochrome P450 isoenzymes (CYP)</u> are minimally involved in the process, which limits the potential of rivastigmine to interact with other drugs and substances metabolised by the CYP system.[18]

> The major CYP isoenzymes are minimally involved in the metabolism of rivastigmine, which limits its drug interaction potential.

Special treatment groups

Due to increased exposure, the dose of rivastigmine should be <u>titrated</u> according to the individual tolerability of patients with <u>renal</u> and mild-to-moderate <u>hepatic</u> impairment.[4] A lack of data precludes the use of rivastigmine in patients with severe hepatic impairment and no pharmacokinetic changes have been reported in patients with severe renal impairment.[4] In summary, no dosage adjustments are necessary when administering rivastigmine to elderly patients, unless they have renal or hepatic impairment, when dose adjustments should be in accordance with tolerability.[4]

> No dosage adjustments are necessary when administering rivastigmine to elderly patients, unless they have renal or <u>hepatic</u> impairment.

Clinical efficacy

A number of investigational tools are routinely used to assess the effectiveness of antidementia drugs in a controlled setting. <u>Cognitive</u> function is commonly assessed with the Alzheimer's Disease Assessment

Scale-cognitive subscale (ADAS-cog) scored out of 70, and the MMSE, scored out of 30. Global functioning uses the Clinical Interview Based Impression of Change (CIBIC), CIBIC-plus and Clinical Global Impression of Change (CGIC) scales and assigns a 1–7 point score, 1, 2, or 3 indicating improvement, 4 denoting no change, and 5, 6 or 7 indicating patient deterioration. The Progressive Deterioration Score (PDS) determines the function and quality of life of the individual patient and the Global Deterioration Score (GDS) broadly measures disease severity according to a number of criteria. Whilst these scales permit the evaluation of an antidementia drug within a clinical trial setting, the limited extent to which they accurately reflect real-life functional changes in a manner that is relevant to patients and their carers, is less than ideal. However, changes of a certain magnitude are generally accepted to correlate with clinically relevant changes (e.g. ≥4 point change on ADAS-cog). Diagnostic inaccuracy, which can be as high as 20%, may further confound data by producing a strong bias in favour of non-response to treatment in Alzheimer's disease.[3]

> Diagnostic inaccuracy may confound data by producing a strong bias in favour of non-response to treatment in Alzheimer's disease.

Placebo-controlled studies

A number of placebo-controlled studies have evaluated the effectiveness of rivastigmine in patients with mild-to-moderate Alzheimer's disease.[19–23] However, the primary clinical evidence supporting the use of rivastigmine in such a patient population is derived from two large studies and one supportive study that formed part of the clinical development programme of the drug. Data from these trials are discussed in more detail below.[19–21] In terms of the effects of rivastigmine on disease progression, the Investigation in the Delay to Diagnosis of Alzheimer's Dementia with Exelon (InDDEx) study is still ongoing, but when completed, will represent the largest placebo-controlled trial of rivastigmine completed to date (n=1010).[24]

One of the pivotal trials included 725 patients with probable mild-to-moderate Alzheimer's disease, defined according to criteria set out by the Diagnostic and Statistical Manual of Mental Disorders, fourth edition (DSM-IV). Patients received low (1–4 mg/day) or high (6–12 mg/day) doses of rivastigmine, or placebo for a period of 26 weeks.[19] Doses were escalated in fixed-weekly increments of 1.5 mg/day over the first 12 weeks of treatment and were maintained for the remaining 14 weeks of the study. At study endpoint, the mean dose of rivastigmine was 10.4 mg/day in the high-dose group and 3.7 mg/day in the low-dose group.

Over the course of the study, cognitive function, measured using the ADAS-cog subscale, declined progressively in the placebo and low-dose rivastigmine groups but improved significantly in the high-dose rivastigmine treatment group (–1.41, –1.24 and +1.17 points, for placebo, low- and high-dose rivastigmine, respectively; $p<0.05$ vs placebo [Figure 2]). The proportion of patients exhibiting a clinically meaningful improvement in their ADAS-cog scores by the end of the study – defined as an improvement of 4 points or more from baseline – was

> Cognitive function declined progressively in the placebo and low-dose rivastigmine groups but improved significantly in the high-dose rivastigmine treatment group.

Figure 2. The mean change from baseline in ADAS-cog (top) and PDS scores (bottom) following 26 weeks of treatment with low- (1–4 mg/day) or high- (6–12 mg/day) dose rivastigmine or placebo.[19] ADAS-cog, Alzheimer's Disease Assessment Scale-cognitive subscale; PDS, Progressive Deterioration Scale.

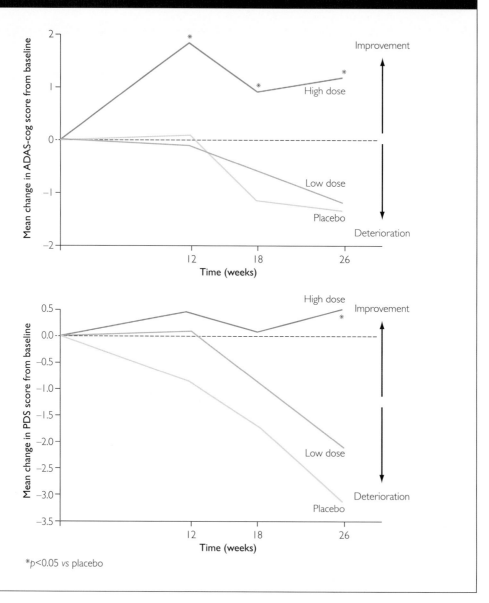

*p<0.05 vs placebo

significantly greater in the high-dose rivastigmine treatment group than in the placebo group (29, 17 and 19% for high dose, low dose and placebo, respectively; p<0.05 vs placebo). Changes in the CIBIC scale over the course of the study followed a similar trend with patients treated in the high-dose rivastigmine group showing significant improvements compared with placebo-treated patients (mean rating 3.93 [indicating improvement] vs 4.34 [indicating no change], for high dose and placebo respectively; $p<0.05$). The mean rating of 4.20 in the low-dose rivastigmine group did not differ significantly from placebo ($p>0.05$). PDS scores were derived from data provided by the caregiver (Figure 2). Only the high-dose rivastigmine treatment group showed significant improvement in PDS score from baseline compared with placebo ($p<0.05$). The study completion rate was 80%, and the discontinuation rate was higher in the high-dose treatment group than in the low-dose or placebo groups (33, 14 and 13% for high dose, low dose and placebo, respectively; p-values not reported). The most common reasons for treatment discontinuation were adverse events (23, 7 and 7%, respectively; p-values not reported), the most common of which were nausea, vomiting, dizziness, headache and diarrhoea.

The other major placebo-controlled trial of rivastigmine was in 699 patients with probable mild-to-moderate Alzheimer's disease, defined using DSM-IV criteria.[20] Participants had an MMSE score between 10 and 26 and had undergone a computed tomography (CT) or magnetic resonance imaging (MRI) scan within 12 months of enrolment into the study and whose results were consistent with Alzheimer's disease. The rivastigmine dosage regimens were identical to those in the study described previously, with the exception that dose escalation occurred over the first 7 rather than the initial 12 weeks of the 26-week study. By the end of the study, the mean dose of rivastigmine was 9.7 mg/day in the higher dose group and 3.5 mg/day in the lower dose group. The frequency of discontinuations closely reflected that in the previously described placebo-controlled trial, with 78% of patients completing their course of treatment. Again, the discontinuation rate was higher in the high-dose treatment group than in the low-dose or placebo groups (35, 15 and 17% for high dose, low dose and placebo, respectively; p-values not reported). The primary reason for treatment discontinuation was intolerable adverse events, which accounted for over 80% of withdrawals from the high-dose treatment group and approximately half of the withdrawals from the low-dose or placebo groups. The most common adverse events reported over the course of the trial were gastrointestinal in nature (e.g. nausea, vomiting, diarrhoea, anorexia) and were mild-to-moderate in intensity. After 26 weeks of treatment, significant therapeutic benefit over placebo was observed in the high-dose rivastigmine treatment group in terms of the ADAS-cog, CIBIC-plus, PDS and GDS scales (Table 2; $p<0.01–0.001$). The low dose of rivastigmine, whilst not as clinically effective as the higher dose with regard to the majority of these evaluations, still elicited significant improvements in ADAS-cog and CIBIC-plus scores compared with placebo at weeks 18 and/or 26 (ADAS-cog: –2.27 vs –4.15; CIBIC-plus: 0.16 vs 0.48; $p<0.05$ vs placebo for both evaluations at week 26).

A 26-week, open-label extension of this study allocated rivastigmine to those patients who completed the study and who were willing to continue with active treatment (n=532).[25] All patients then received rivastigmine at a dose of 1 mg twice daily for the first week irrespective of prior treatment allocation. Thereafter, the dose of rivastigmine was increased or reduced according to the individual's tolerability, up to a

Table 2. Primary outcome measures after 26 weeks of treatment with high- or low-dose rivastigmine or placebo (observed case analysis).[20]

Treatment (n)	Outcome measures			
	ADAS-cog	CIBIC-plus	PDS	GDS
High-dose rivastigmine (n=145)	0.79	0.13	−1.15	−0.14
Low-dose rivastigmine (n=194)	−2.27	0.16	−5.25	−0.15
Placebo (n=192)	−4.15	0.48	−5.69	−0.33
Treatment difference (high dose vs placebo)	4.94	−0.35	4.54	0.19
p-value	<0.001	<0.01	<0.001	<0.012

ADAS-cog, Alzheimer's Disease Assessment Scale-cognitive subscale; CIBIC-plus, Clinical Interview Based Impression of Change; GDS, Global Deterioration Score; PDS, Progressive Deterioration Score.

maximum of 6 mg, twice daily. The percentage of patients achieving a mean rivastigmine dose of 6–12 mg/day at week 52 was 72% in the original 6–12 mg/day treatment group, 68% in the original 1–4 mg/day treatment group and 65% amongst those patients who originally received placebo. The effect of continued (or newly initiated) treatment with rivastigmine on ADAS-cog scores is shown in Figure 3. The greatest improvement in ADAS-cog was observed in those patients who originally received high-dose rivastigmine (greater than 4 points improvement reported in 15, 6 and 8% of original high-dose, low-dose and placebo groups respectively; *p*=0.085 high dose *vs* placebo). Over the course of this open-label extension, approximately 97% patients reported at least one adverse event. Consistent with the original study, the most common adverse events reported were gastrointestinal (e.g. nausea, vomiting, diarrhoea and anorexia).

These placebo-controlled studies and their open-label extensions have formed the basis for further analyses, which have:

- highlighted the sustained benefits achieved by early intervention with rivastigmine treatment
- demonstrated a potential delaying effect of rivastigmine on disease progression
- identified factors predictive of treatment success with rivastigmine (e.g. rapid cognitive decline or more severe disease at baseline).[26–30]

Patients with more rapidly progressing Alzheimer's disease continue to progress at a rapid rate throughout their disease, enter severe stages of disease sooner and die earlier.[31] In order to test whether the response to rivastigmine treatment varied according to the severity of Alzheimer's disease, patients from placebo-controlled studies[19–21] were stratified according to severity of their dementia (mild, moderate or severe).[30] It was found that treatment with rivastigmine (6–12 mg/day) maintained

Figure 3. The mean change from baseline in Alzheimer's Disease Assessment Scale-cognitive subscale (ADAS-cog) score following 52 weeks of treatment with low- (1–4 mg/day) or high- (6–12 mg/day) dose rivastigmine or placebo.[25]

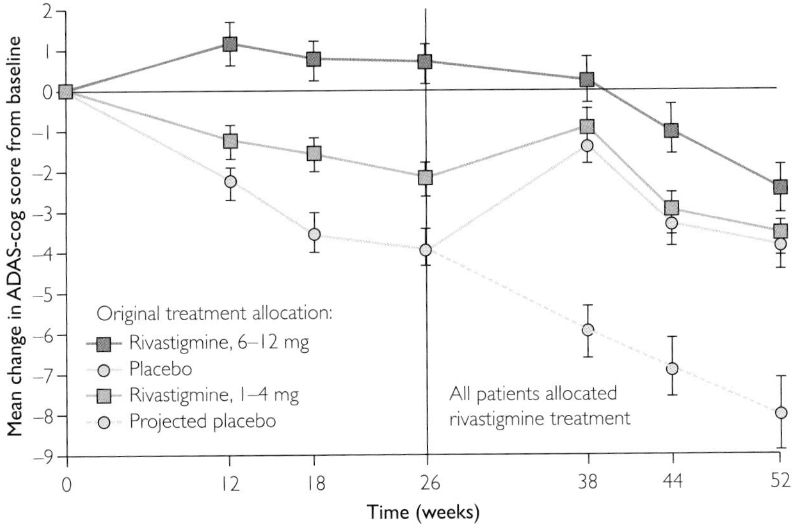

ADAS-cog scores at or above placebo levels in all severity cohorts, whereas cognitive deterioration with placebo was progressive and severity dependent. The strongest effects of rivastigmine were observed in patients with moderate or moderately severe Alzheimer's disease and may, at least partly, be a consequence of its dual inhibition of acetyl- and butyrylcholinesterase.[30]

A further retrospective analysis of pooled data from placebo-controlled trials[19–21] selectively examined patients with more severe cognitive impairment (10–12 MMSE points, n=117).[32] It was found that after 6 months, the mean ADAS-cog score had declined by 6.3 points in the placebo groups, but increased by 0.2 points in the rivastigmine treatment group ($p<0.001$). Interestingly, the relative risk of discontinuing treatment prematurely as a result of intolerable adverse events was lower than in participants with milder disease (relative risk 2.0 *vs* 3.6, respectively).

Of the acetylcholinesterase inhibitors investigated to date, only rivastigmine has demonstrated a preferential effect in patients with rapid disease progression.

> Of the acetylcholinesterase inhibitors investigated to date, only rivastigmine has demonstrated a preferential effect in patients with rapid disease progression.

Meta-analyses

A pooled analysis of three placebo-controlled studies of rivastigmine, all of 26 weeks' duration, included a total of 2126 patients, 1479 of whom received rivastigmine.[21] For two of the trials (described previously), the dosage regimens were flexible, with patients receiving either low (1–4 mg/day) or high (6–12 mg/day) doses of rivastigmine.[19,20] In the other 'supportive' study, which was published only as part of this pooled analysis, the dose of rivastigmine was fixed at either 3, 6 or 9 mg/day, following initial dose titration.[21] Aside from these differences in dose schedules, the baseline demographics of patients were comparable in the different studies. Overall, rivastigmine-treated patients showed significant improvements in cognition, function and activities of daily living, as determined by using the ADAS-cog, CIBIC and PDS scales of assessment, respectively (Table 3 and Figure 4).

A further meta-analysis evaluated data derived from four 6-month placebo-controlled trials of rivastigmine, which also included open-label drug treatment, up to 12 mg/day, given for a total treatment period of up to 5 years.[33] The effects of rivastigmine were compared with the projected cognitive decline of untreated patients over the same period. At baseline, MMSE data were available for 1998 rivastigmine-treated patients, and the mean baseline MMSE score was 19.3. After 5 years, 83 patients remained on rivastigmine therapy. The model-based curve for untreated patients showed a decline in MMSE score to below the threshold of 12 points after approximately 2.5 years, whereas the mean rivastigmine curve remained above 12 points after 5 years of treatment. Therefore, rivastigmine appears to prevent the decline to severe dementia (MMSE score of less than 10 points) by at least 2 years.

The rate of cognitive decline amongst rivastigmine-treated patients was also assessed over 2 years, in a pooled analysis of four 6-month placebo-controlled studies and two open-label extension studies

> Rivastigmine appears to prevent the decline to severe dementia by at least 2 years.

Table 3. Items on the Progressive Deterioration Scale (PDS) showing significant improvement following treatment with rivastigmine (6–12 mg/day).[21]

PDS item	Percentage of patients showing clinically meaningful improvement[a]		p-value
	Rivastigmine (6–12 mg/day)	Placebo	
Stops family finances	26	21	0.029
Drives car	28	20	<0.001
Discusses politics	30	23	0.010
Stops household chores	28	23	0.03
Cannot handle money	28	22	0.007
Confusion in different settings	33	27	0.010
Forgets things	34	25	<0.001
Rearranges objects	32	24	<0.001
Dresses properly	26	18	<0.001
Cannot use telephone	27	20	<0.001
Walks safely	25	20	0.018

[a] ≥10% improvement

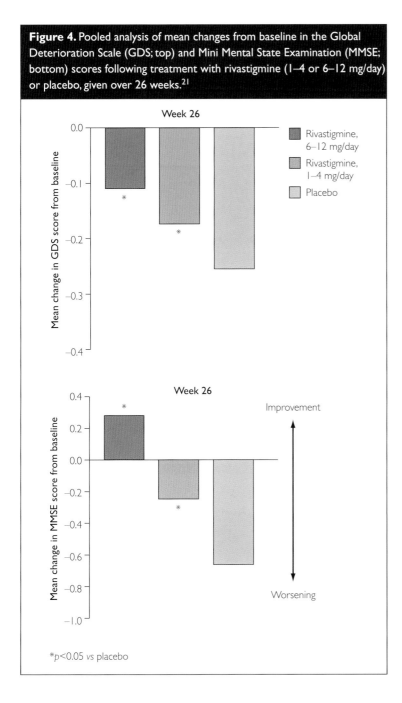

Figure 4. Pooled analysis of mean changes from baseline in the Global Deterioration Scale (GDS; top) and Mini Mental State Examination (MMSE; bottom) scores following treatment with rivastigmine (1–4 or 6–12 mg/day) or placebo, given over 26 weeks.[21]

(n=2010).[34] Cognitive deterioration was less pronounced following treatment with rivastigmine compared with untreated historical-controls (change in ADAS-cog score: 8.6 *vs* 11.6 for rivastigmine-treated patients and untreated controls, respectively; *p-value* not reported). According to caregiver and clinician assessments, these findings regarding cognitive performance were of a sufficient magnitude as to be relevant to global patient functioning.[34]

Behavioural and psychological symptoms of dementia (BPSD) are amongst the most distressing manifestations of Alzheimer's disease.[35] BPSD affect up to 80% of patients with Alzheimer's disease and contribute considerably to its social and economic burden. In this respect, they are often the single largest factor in the decision to institutionalise patients.[35] Whilst all acetylcholinesterase inhibitors have been shown to improve apathy, depression and anxiety, only rivastigmine has demonstrated additional improvement in hallucinations and delusions. This may be a consequence of its dual inhibition of acetyl- and butyrylcholinesterase.[35] It has also been proposed that the presence of hallucinations may even predict a positive response to rivastigmine therapy.[35] The success of rivastigmine in relieving hallucinations may reflect its ability to enhance Rapid Eye Movement (REM) sleep, which is know to have a cholinergic basis.[36]

A meta-analysis of three 6-month, placebo-controlled, regulatory trials of rivastigmine in patients with mild-to-moderate Alzheimer's disease, stratified patients (n=1840) according to the presence or absence of disruptive BPSD at baseline, in order to determine the effects of rivastigmine upon behavioural symptoms of Alzheimer's disease.[37] Overall, treatment with rivastigmine, 6–12 mg/day, was shown to improve or prevent disruptive BPSD ($p<0.05$ *vs* placebo). Patients with behavioural symptoms at baseline showed significant improvement in paranoid and delusional ideation and aggressiveness compared with placebo (improvement observed in 60 *vs* 48% and 54 *vs* 45% of rivastigmine- and placebo-treated patients for paranoia and aggressiveness, respectively; $p=0.001$ and $p=0.046$). Rivastigmine also appeared to prevent the emergence of activity disturbances compared with placebo (22.5 *vs* 32.5% for rivastigmine and placebo, respectively; $p=0.016$). The findings of this meta-analysis may account for the reduced use of antipsychotic agents amongst rivastigmine-treated patients (see Safety and Tolerability), of particular relevance following the Committee on Safety of Medicines (CSM) restriction on the prescribing of risperidone and olanzapine to elderly patients with dementia owing to the risk of cerebrovascular adverse events.

To summarise, the placebo-controlled studies of rivastigmine in patients with mild-to-moderate Alzheimer's disease have demonstrated the following observations.

- Significant improvements from baseline in ADAS-cog scores over 26 weeks following high-dose rivastigmine treatment (6–12 mg/day), that appear to be sustainable for up to 1 year.
- Significant improvement from baseline in CIBIC scores over 26 weeks following high-dose rivastigmine treatment, compared with placebo.
- Significant improvement from baseline in PDS scores over 26 weeks following high-dose rivastigmine treatment, compared with placebo.
- The lower dose of rivastigmine (1–4 mg/day)[b] was less effective than the higher dose. However, limited improvements in ADAS-cog and

> Treatment with rivastigmine, 6–12 mg/day, was shown to improve or prevent disruptive BPSD.

---

[b]Not licensed.

CIBIC-plus scores were reported in one study following low-dose rivastigmine.

- Treatment with rivastigmine (6–12 mg/day) was shown to improve or prevent disruptive BPSD, compared with placebo.
- The majority of patients in these studies persisted with rivastigmine treatment, with a completion rate of approximately 80%. Adverse events were the primary reason for treatment discontinuation and were predominantly gastrointestinal in nature.

Open-label studies

Post-marketing surveillance

An open-label, post-marketing surveillance study conducted across Germany, examined the effectiveness of rivastigmine over 12 months in 1302 patients with mild-to-moderately severe Alzheimer's disease.[38] At baseline, the mean daily dosage of rivastigmine was 3.3 mg, which increased to 5.7 mg after 3 months and 6.9 mg after 1 year. Symptoms were evaluated by the physician and after 3 months of treatment with rivastigmine, 92% patients were rated as unchanged or improved. At 1 year, 82% of patients were unchanged or improved, with the remaining 18% showing significant signs of disease progression. Caregivers reported a slightly lower need for care over the year of treatment, with 50.1% of patients requiring no care at all at baseline, compared with 58.3% at the study endpoint. Rivastigmine was well tolerated and 87.9% patients showed no adverse events over the course of the investigation.

Rivastigmine vs donepezil

The therapeutic benefits of treatment with either rivastigmine or donepezil were compared in an open-label study in 111 patients with mild-to-moderate Alzheimer's disease.[39] Over the 12 weeks of the study, patients received either rivastigmine, up to 6 mg twice daily, or donepezil, up to 10 mg twice daily. The rate of study completion was significantly higher in the donepezil treatment group (89.3 vs 69.1%, for donepezil and rivastigmine, respectively; p=0.009). The rate of discontinuation as a result of intolerable adverse events was higher amongst rivastigmine-treated patients (21.8 vs 10.7%, respectively; p-value not reported). However, the 2-week rivastigmine dose-titration interval employed may have adversely affected its tolerability and may account for the comparatively high discontinuation rate amongst rivastigmine-treated participants.[40] In terms of clinical efficacy, improvements from baseline on the ADAS-cog scale (rated by blinded, independent observers) were comparable between the two treatment groups at weeks 4 and 12 (–2.02 vs –2.14 at week 4 and –1.05 vs –0.90 at week 12, for rivastigmine and donepezil, respectively; p-value not reported). These data show that whilst donepezil appeared to be better tolerated, the two drugs elicited similar levels of improvement in cognitive function. The relevance of this study to clinical practice is disputable, not least because of its short-term nature.

Switching between cholinesterase inhibitors

Accumulated evidence suggests that switching between cholinesterase inhibitors may evoke a positive treatment response in patients who had previously failed to respond to their original drug therapy, either as a result of a lack of efficacy, a loss of efficacy or safety and tolerability issues.[41] When treating Alzheimer's disease, it is important to persist for a minimum of 6 months with an initial treatment before considering switching to an alternative agent, and the decision to switch must be based on realistic treatment expectations.[41]

An open-label, 6-month study examined the effect of switching to rivastigmine (up to 12 mg/day) in 382 patients with Alzheimer's disease who had previously failed to demonstrate benefit following at least 6 months of treatment with donepezil (5–10 mg/day).[42] Patients had discontinued donepezil at least 7 days before beginning rivastigmine treatment. Eighty per cent of patients had withdrawn from donepezil treatment as a result of a lack of efficacy, 11% due to tolerability issues and 9% for a combination of both reasons. Lack of efficacy was defined as at least a 2-point decrease in MMSE score within 12 months of treatment initiation, or a significant decrease in functional autonomy. At baseline, the mean MMSE score was 16.6. After 6 months of treatment with rivastigmine, the mean improvement in MMSE score from baseline was 0.9 points ($p<0.001$ vs baseline) amongst those patients rated as responders on the CGIC scale (56.2% of the total study population). In contrast, CGIC non-responders (43.9% of the study population) showed a mean deterioration of –2.7 points on the MMSE scale (p-value not reported). Although 48.9% of patients experienced at least a 1-point improvement or stabilisation in MMSE score compared with baseline, the overall mean change from baseline across all patients was –0.7 points, indicative of cognitive decline (p-value not reported). Over 80% of patients completed the study, with adverse events (e.g. nausea, vomiting, agitation, weight loss and anorexia) the most common reason for early treatment discontinuation (11% of patients), with a lack of efficacy responsible for 1.8% of participants withdrawing from the study. Overall, a lack of response to donepezil treatment was not an accurate predictor of similar problems with rivastigmine and switching treatments led to a positive response in approximately 50% of patients.

> Lack of response to donepezil treatment was not an accurate predictor of similar problems with rivastigmine and switching treatments led to a positive response in approximately 50% of patients.

Patients with Alzheimer's disease and concurrent hypertension

Data derived from a 15-year longitudinal study suggest that previously increased blood pressure may increase the risk for dementia by inducing small-vessel disease and white-matter lesions.[43] Two separate analyses have stratified patients from the two major placebo-controlled studies of rivastigmine on the basis of their vascular risk.

Patients from the <u>placebo-controlled</u> study by Corey-Bloom *et al.*,[20] were grouped according to their Modified Hachinski Ischaemic Score (MHIS), the criteria of which include abrupt onset of <u>dementia</u>, <u>stepwise deterioration</u> of the patient, <u>somatic</u> complaints, emotional incontinence, history of stroke, <u>focal neurological</u> signs and a history or presence of <u>hypertension</u>.[20,44] At <u>baseline</u>, 378 patients had an MHIS score of zero whilst 319 had an MHIS score greater than zero. Patients with scores above five were excluded as their <u>vascular</u> risk was inconsistent with probable Alzheimer's disease.[44] The study completion rate was comparable between MHIS subgroups (78 *vs* 79% for MHIS zero and MHIS>zero, respectively). The changes from baseline in <u>ADAS-cog</u> scores were significantly different, with the vascular risk factor group (MHIS>zero) showing greater therapeutic benefit than the non-risk group (treatment difference of 2.3 points; $p=0.02$ [Figure 5]). There were no major differences in the type or nature of <u>adverse events</u> between the two MHIS groups.

In a similar analysis, the 725 patients from the placebo-controlled study by Rösler *et al.*,[19] were stratified according to MHIS score and the presence or absence of arterial hypertension at baseline, defined as blood pressure greater than 160/100 mmHg.[19,45] At baseline, 24.6% of the total study population were hypertensive (22, 24 and 28% of the <u>placebo</u>, low and high dose rivastigmine treatment groups, respectively). Study completion rates were generally comparable between hypertensive and non-hypertensive patients (88 *vs* 87%, 81 *vs* 89% and 70 *vs* 69% in placebo, low and high dose groups, respectively; <u>*p*-values</u> not reported).

> The changes from baseline in <u>ADAS-cog</u> scores were significantly different, with the vascular risk factor group showing greater therapeutic benefit than the non-risk group.

Figure 5. The mean change from baseline in Alzheimer's Disease Assessment Scale-cognitive subscale (ADAS-cog) score following 26 weeks of treatment with rivastigmine (1–4 mg/day or 6–12 mg/day) or placebo. Patients stratified according to Modified Hachinski Ischaemic Score (MHIS).[44]

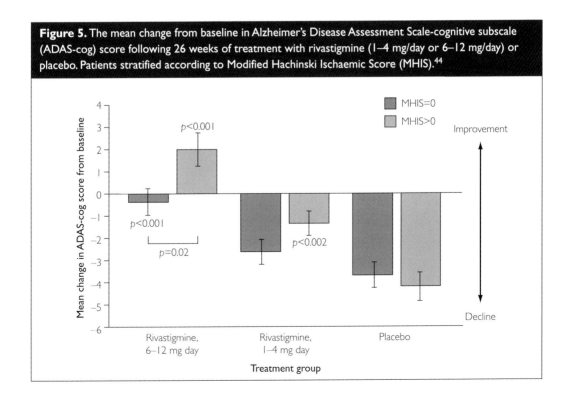

Overall treatment differences between hypertensive and non-hypertensive patients, in terms of ADAS-cog scores, were non-significant across the high dose group ($p=0.185$). However, significantly more hypertensive than non-hypertensive patients showed improvements on the ADAS-cog items of word recognition ($p<0.05$) and orientation ($p<0.01$) following high-dose rivastigmine treatment. No differences were detected between placebo and low-dose rivastigmine on the basis of hypertensive status. Aside from a lower incidence of nausea and vomiting amongst rivastigmine-treated patients with hypertension than in those without, the nature and frequency of adverse events was unaffected by hypertensive status. Additionally, no cardiac adverse events or clinically significant drug–drug interactions were reported.

An open-label extension of the study by Rösler *et al.*,[19] examined the long-term efficacy of rivastigmine over a period of 2 years.[19,46] All patients entering the extension received individually tailored rivastigmine treatment (2–12 mg/day). Those patients having received rivastigmine for the whole duration of the trial (n=162) were termed 'early starters' and those patients who initially received placebo (n=178) were termed 'late starters'. After 104 weeks, all patients showed deterioration in ADAS-cog scores from baseline, although the decline amongst hypertensive early starters was approximately half that in hypertensive late starters (3.28 *vs* 7.04 points for early and late starters respectively; $p=0.077$). Amongst non-hypertensive patients, changes from baseline ADAS-cog at week 104 were unaffected by the time point at which rivastigmine treatment was initiated (7.3 *vs* 7.6 points for early and late starters, respectively; $p>0.05$). The changes from baseline in PDS scores are illustrated in Figure 6 (week 104: –8.96 *vs* –20.52 points for early and late starters respectively; $p=0.013$).

Taken together, these data suggest that patients with vascular risk factors may experience greater clinical benefit from rivastigmine, in terms of cognitive improvement, global functioning and quality of life, and that these differences may be sustained in the long-term (up to 2 years). It has been proposed that the additional benefit that rivastigmine confers to hypertensive patients may be linked to the effect the drug has on cerebrovascular factors. Preclinical studies have demonstrated a protective action of rivastigmine in ischaemic brain conditions and increased cerebral blood flow due to rivastigmine, of particular relevance considering that patients with Alzheimer's disease have been shown to have impaired cerebral blood flow.[44]

Safety and tolerability

Data derived from controlled clinical trials show that the majority of adverse events associated with rivastigmine are gastrointestinal (e.g. nausea, vomiting, diarrhoea) and are dose-related, mild or moderate in severity and transient in nature (Figure 7).[47] Treatment-related adverse events represent the most common reason for therapy discontinuation amongst patients with Alzheimer's disease. There is some evidence to suggest that women are particularly susceptible to the gastrointestinal

Figure 6. The mean change from baseline in the Progressive Deterioration Scale (PDS) in hypertensive and non-hypertensive patients over 104 weeks.[46]

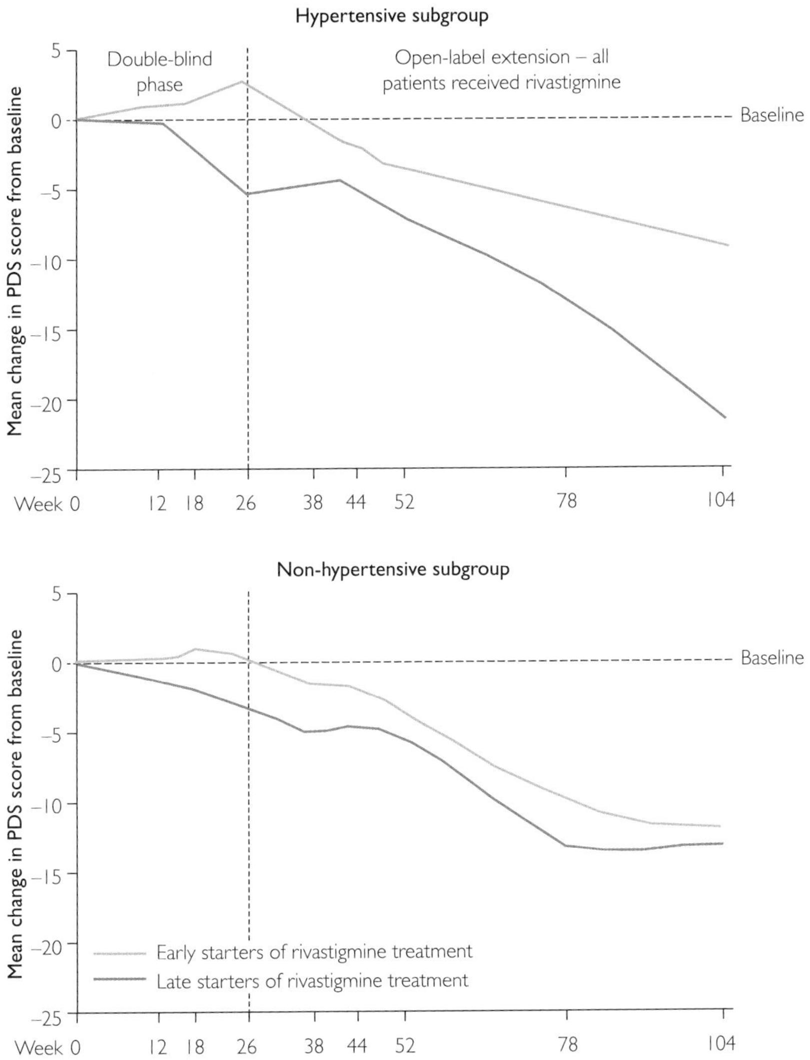

side-effects associated with rivastigmine, although the reasons for this are unclear.[4] Other commonly reported side-effects include dyspepsia, anorexia, abdominal pain, dizziness, headache, drowsiness, tremor, asthenia, malaise, agitation and confusion.[17] In contrast to donepezil, treatment with rivastigmine is not commonly associated with extra-pyramidal symptoms, muscle stiffness, slowness of movement or postural instability, possibly due to a relative lack of G4 acetylcholinesterase inhibition in the striatum.[48] Bradycardia, sleep disturbances and urinary

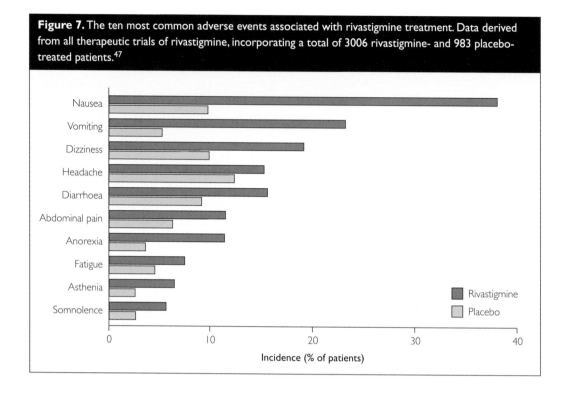

Figure 7. The ten most common adverse events associated with rivastigmine treatment. Data derived from all therapeutic trials of rivastigmine, incorporating a total of 3006 rivastigmine- and 983 placebo-treated patients.[47]

symptoms are also less commonly associated with rivastigmine than donepezil treatment.[49] The <u>adverse event</u> rate may be reduced by slowing the dose escalation of rivastigmine, leaving a minimum of 4 weeks between dose increments, and if gastrointestinal effects are particularly restrictive, patients may respond to omitting one or more doses.[4,18,48]

The response to rivastigmine treatment (up to 12 mg/day) in clinical practice was assessed in 529 outpatients with mild-to-moderate Alzheimer's disease in Austria over a 24-week treatment period.[50] Eighty-seven per cent of patients completed the study and of the 13% of patients who did not, 40.3% experienced adverse events, although it is not clear whether this was the main reason for treatment discontinuation. Overall, 33.8% patients experienced a total of 305 adverse events, the majority of which were mild or moderate and transient, and predominantly involved the gastrointestinal system (30.4%). Nausea was the most common and affected 16.8% patients, the next most frequent was vertigo (5.3%), vomiting (4.9%), loss of appetite (3.2%), tiredness (2.5%), weight loss (1.7%), headache (1.5%) and tremor (1.5%). Physicians judged that 62.1% of study participants responded very well or well to treatment together with very good-to-good drug tolerability.

The analysis of pooled electrocardiographic (ECG) data from the <u>placebo-controlled</u> trials of rivastigmine, encompassing a total of 2791 patients, revealed no significant drug-related effects on heart rate, PR interval, corrected QT interval or QRS complex after 26 weeks of rivastigmine treatment.[51]

Rivastigmine is associated with a low incidence of adverse sleep effects in patients with Alzheimer's disease.[49] Compared with donepezil, rivastigmine showed lower potential for abnormal dreams (1.9 vs 7.1% for rivastigmine and donepezil, respectively; p-value not reported) in an open-label comparative study.[39] Furthermore, direct sleep studies have shown that treatment with rivastigmine increased REM density without affecting REM latency, suggesting minimal disturbance of brainstem function.[48,49]

> Rivastigmine is associated with a low incidence of adverse sleep effects in patients with Alzheimer's disease.

Special warnings and precautions

Rivastigmine should be used with caution in patients with:
- renal impairment
- mild-to-moderate hepatic impairment
- sick sinus syndrome or conduction defects (sino-atrial block, atrio-ventricular block)
- active gastric or duodenal ulcers
- a history of asthma or pulmonary disease
- a predisposition to urinary obstructions or seizures
- Parkinson's disease (may induce or exacerbate extrapyramidal symptoms).[4]

Drug interactions

In view of its independence from metabolism by liver microsomal enzymes and its limited plasma protein binding, rivastigmine is unlikely to be involved in significant interactions with other medications. However, there is some evidence that rivastigmine may exacerbate the effects of succinylcholine-type muscle relaxants during anaesthesia (e.g. suxamethonium) and it should not be given concomitantly with other cholinomimetic drugs.[4]

The analysis of data from placebo-controlled trials incorporating a total of 2459 patients, detected no serious adverse pharmacodynamic drug interactions between rivastigmine and 22 classes of medication including antacids, diabetes drugs, α- and β-adrenoceptor blocking agents, calcium-channel blockers, diuretics, anti-inflammatory drugs, anti-emetics and angiotensin-converting enzymes (ACE) inhibitors.[52]

Use of antipsychotic medication

Many patients with Alzheimer's disease may be prescribed antipsychotics in order to control some of the behavioural symptoms associated with the disorder. As mentioned previously, clinical data suggest that rivastigmine may limit the need for antipsychotic medication, a particularly pertinent finding in light of the recent CSM restriction on the prescribing of risperidone and olanzapine to elderly patients with dementia.[53,54] An analysis of data from Alzheimer's disease patients prescribed rivastigmine who had not used antipsychotic medication within the 18 months prior to diagnosis or prescription (n=497), compared subsequent antipsychotic usage with patients not receiving anticholinesterase treatment (n=749).[54] The overall use of antipsychotics (typical [e.g. chlorpromazine, haloperidol, loxapine] or atypical [e.g. clozapine, olanzapine, risperidone]) was higher amongst untreated patients (25.6 *vs* 9.8%; no *p*-value reported). Treatment with rivastigmine delayed the use of antipsychotic use compared with patients not taking cholinesterase inhibitors (relative risk 0.36; $p<0.001$). This study implies that rivastigmine treatment could delay the onset of behavioural symptoms that necessitate the use of antipsychotics in patients with Alzheimer's disease.

Pharmacoeconomics

The cost of Alzheimer's disease increases with disease severity and the financial implications of increased hours of care by the caregiver increase proportionally.[55] It is estimated that by improving cognitive function and slowing the rate of cognitive decline, cholinesterase inhibitors may reduce the economic burden of Alzheimer's disease by delaying the patient's progression to a nursing home setting.

The effect of rivastigmine on the financial burden of Alzheimer's disease has been examined in a number of studies, although long-term prospective data are currently lacking in this area.[56–58] A review of these studies revealed that, excluding drug acquisition costs, treatment with rivastigmine reduced the economic consequences of disease in patients with mild-to-moderate Alzheimer's disease by increasing the time elapsed before institutionalisation became necessary.[59] If the cost of rivastigmine was factored in then the cost-saving partially or completely offset treatment acquisition costs. The largest savings were in patients with mild disease treated over a 2-year period, thus highlighting the importance of early initiation of rivastigmine treatment from an economic perspective.

Analyses of the comparative cost-effectiveness of rivastigmine, donepezil and galantamine are hampered by difficulties encountered when comparing data derived from different sources which employ different outcome parameters and methodology.[60,61] The use of Markov models, with different transition probabilities, and hazard models of cognitive decline, makes comparisons difficult. Thus, potential cost-savings attributable to rivastigmine over donepezil or galantamine cannot be accurately determined on the basis of current data.

Key points

- Rivastigmine is a centrally selective <u>pseudo-irreversible</u> <u>cholinesterase inhibitor</u> indicated for the symptomatic treatment of mild-to-moderate Alzheimer's disease.

- By inhibiting the degradation of <u>acetylcholine</u> by the acetyl- and <u>butyrylcholinesterase</u> <u>enzymes</u>, rivastigmine improves <u>cholinergic</u> function and shows benefit on <u>cognitive</u>, global and ADL functions in Alzheimer's disease.

- The inhibition of butyrylcholinesterase is unique to rivastigmine since donepezil and galantamine only inhibit <u>acetylcholinesterase</u>.

- The pharmacodynamic <u>mechanism of action</u> of rivastigmine supports twice-daily dosing.

- Since rivastigmine is not metabolised by CYP enzymes and also has limited binding to plasma proteins, it shows limited propensity for clinically relevant <u>drug–drug</u> <u>interactions</u> and may be co-administered with a large number of other medications.

- In <u>placebo-controlled</u> clinical trials, rivastigmine elicited significant improvements in cognitive and global measures of clinical change and slowed the rate of deterioration of patients with mild-to-moderate Alzheimer's disease compared with <u>placebo</u>.

- Long-term, <u>open-label</u> extension studies of rivastigmine have demonstrated continued clinical benefits after up to 5 years of treatment.

- Rivastigmine treatment has been shown to improve or prevent disruptive BPSD, which may account for the reduced use of anti-psychotic medication associated with the drug.

- One study demonstrated that a high proportion of patients who could not tolerate or did not benefit from treatment with donepezil treatment, responded well to rivastigmine treatment.

- Patients with <u>cardiovascular</u> risk factors may experience greater therapeutic benefit from rivastigmine treatment than normotensive patients with Alzheimer's disease.

- Rivastigmine is associated with a dose-related increase in the frequency of gastrointestinal <u>adverse events</u>, which are usually mild-to-moderate in severity and resolve with continued treatment.

Any reference made to guidance from the National Institute of Clinical Excellence (NICE) in the preceding section relates to guidelines published in 2001. As we go to press (March 2005), NICE has issued preliminary guidance that is currently under review and will be finalised and published later in 2005 (see Editor's notes Pages xx and 127).

References

A list of the published evidence which has been reviewed in compiling the preceding section of *BESTMEDICINE.*

1 Scarpini E, Scheltens P, Feldman H. Treatment of Alzheimer's disease: current status and new perspectives. *Lancet Neurol* 2003; **2**: 539–47.

2 Williams B, Nazarians A, Gill M. A review of rivastigmine: a reversible cholinesterase inhibitor. *Clin Ther* 2003; **25**: 1634–53.

3 Francis P, Palmer A, Snape M, Wilcock G. The cholinergic hypothesis of Alzheimer's disease: a review of progress. *J Neurol Neurosurg Psychiatry.* 1998; **66**: 137–47.

4 *Exelon® (Rivastigmine). Summary of Product Characteristics.* Novartis Ltd., 2003.

5 National Institute for Clinical Excellence. Guidance on the use of donepezil, rivastigmine and galantamine for the treatment of Alzheimer's disease. Technology Appraisal Guidance. 2001.*www.nice.org.uk*

6 Polinsky R. Clinical pharmacology of rivastigmine: a new-generation acetylcholinesterase inhibitor for the treatment of Alzheimer's disease. *Clin Ther* 1998; **20**: 634–47.

7 Mesulam M, Guillozet A, Shaw P *et al.* Acetylcholinesterase knockouts establish central cholinergic pathways and can use butyrylcholinesterase to hydrolyze acetylcholine. *Neuroscience* 2002; **110**: 627–39.

8 Arendt T, Bruckner M, Lange M, Bigl V. Changes in acetylcholinesterase and butyrylcholinesterase in Alzheimer's disease resemble embryonic development – a study of molecular forms. *Neurochem Int* 1992; **21**: 381–96.

9 Perry E, Perry R, Blessed G, Tomlinson B. Changes in brain cholinesterases in senile dementia of Alzheimer type. *Neuropathol Appl Neurobiol* 1978; **4**: 273–7.

10 Siek G, Katz L, Fishman E, Korosi T, Marquis J. Molecular forms of acetylcholinesterase in subcortical areas of normal and Alzheimer disease brain. *Biol Psychiatry* 1990; **27**: 573–80.

11 Giacobini E, Spiegel R, Enz A, Veroff A, Cutler N. Inhibition of acetyl- and butyryl-cholinesterase in the cerebrospinal fluid of patients with Alzheimer's disease by rivastigmine: correlation with cognitive benefit. *J Neural Transm* 2002; **109**: 1053–65.

12 Almkvist O, Darreh-Shori T, Stefanova E, Spiegel R, Nordberg A. Preserved cognitive function after 12 months of treatment with rivastigmine in mild Alzheimer's disease in comparison with untreated AD and MCI patients. *Eur J Neurol* 2004; **11**: 253–61.

13 Potkin S, Anand R, Fleming K *et al.* Brain metabolic and clinical effects of rivastigmine in Alzheimer's disease. *Int J Neuropsychopharmacol* 2001; **4**: 223–30.

14 Stefanova E, Blennow K, Almkvist O, Hellstrom-Lindahl E, Nordberg A. Cerebral glucose metabolism, cerebrospinal fluid-beta-amyloid1-42 (CSF-Abeta42), tau and apolipoprotein E genotype in long-term rivastigmine and tacrine treated Alzheimer disease (AD) patients. *Neurosci Lett* 2003; **338**: 159–63.

15 Lojkowska W, Ryglewicz D, Jedrzejczak T *et al.* The effect of cholinesterase inhibitors on the regional blood flow in patients with Alzheimer's disease and vascular dementia. *J Neurol Sci* 2003; **216**: 119–26.

16 Hossain M, Jhee S, Shiovitz T *et al.* Estimation of the absolute bioavailability of rivastigmine in patients with mild to moderate dementia of the Alzheimer's type. *Clin Pharmacokinet* 2002; **41**: 225–34.

17 *British National Formulary (BNF) 48.* London: British Medical Association and Royal Pharmaceutical Society of Great Britain. September, 2004.

18 Farlow M. Update on rivastigmine. *Neurologist* 2003; **9**: 230–4.

19 Rosler M, Anand R, Cicin-Sain A *et al.* Efficacy and safety of rivastigmine in patients with Alzheimer's disease: international randomised controlled trial. *BMJ* 1999; **318**: 633–8.

20 Corey-Bloom J, Anand R, Veach J. A randomised trial evaluating the efficacy and safety of ENA-713 (rivastigmine tartrate), a new acetylcholinesterase inhibitor, in patients with mild-to-moderately severe Alzheimer's disease. *Int J Geriatr Psychopharmacol* 1998; **1**: 55–65.

21 Schneider L, Anand R, Farlow M. Systematic review of the efficacy of rivastigmine for patients with Alzheimer's disease. *Int J Geriatr Psychopharmacol* 1998; **1**: S26–34.

22 Adler G, Brassen S, Chwalek K, Dieter B, Teufel M. Prediction of treatment response to rivastigmine in Alzheimer's dementia. *J Neurol Neurosurg Psychiatry.* 2004; **75**: 292–4.

23 Forette F, Anand R, Gharabawi G. A phase II study in patients with Alzheimer's disease to assess the preliminary efficacy and maximum tolerated dose of rivastigmine (Exelon). *Eur J Neurol* 1999; **6**: 423–9.

24 Feldman H, Scheltens P, Scarpini E *et al.* Behavioral symptoms in mild cognitive impairment. *Neurology* 2004; **62**: 1199–201.

25 Farlow M, Anand R, Messina J, Hartman R, Veach J. A 52-week study of the efficacy of rivastigmine in patients with mild to moderately severe Alzheimer's disease. *Eur Neurol* 2000; **44**: 236–41.

26 Doraiswamy P, Krishnan K, Anand R *et al.* Long-term effects of rivastigmine in moderately severe Alzheimer's disease: does early initiation of therapy offer sustained benefits? *Prog Neuropsychopharmacol Biol Psychiatry* 2002; **26**: 705–12.

27 Farlow M, Hake A, Messina J *et al.* Response of patients with Alzheimer disease to rivastigmine treatment is predicted by the rate of disease progression. *Arch Neurol* 2001; **58**: 417–22.

28 Farlow M, Potkin S, Koumaras B, Veach J, Mirski D. Analysis of outcome in retrieved dropout patients in a rivastigmine *vs* placebo, 26-week, Alzheimer disease trial. *Arch Neurol* 2003; **60**: 843–8.

29 Farlow M, Small G, Quarg P. Does rivastigmine provide additional benefits in patients with rapid disease progression? 9th International Conference on Alzheimer's Disease and Related Disorders. Philadelphia, 2004.

30 Kurz A, Farlow M, Quarg P, Spiegel R. Disease stage in Alzheimer disease and treatment effects of rivastigmine. *Alzheimer Dis Assoc Disord* 2004; **18**: 123–8.

31 Doody R, Massman P, Dunn J. A method for estimating progression rates in Alzheimer disease. *Arch Neurol* 2001; **58**: 449–54.

32 Burns A, Spiegel R, Quarg P. Efficacy of rivastigmine in subjects with moderately severe Alzheimer's disease. *Int J Geriatr Psychiatry* 2004; **19**: 243–9.

33 Small G, Mendiondo M, Spiegel R. *Efficacy of rivastigmine treatment in Alzheimer's disease over 5 years. 42nd American College of Neuropsychopharmacology Annual Meeting.* San Juan, Puerto Rico, 2003.

34 Grossberg G, Irwin P, Satlin A, Mesenbrink P, Spiegel R. Rivastigmine in Alzheimer disease: efficacy over two years. *Am J Geriatr Psychiatry* 2004; **12**: 420–31.

35 Robert P. Understanding and managing behavioural symptoms in Alzheimer's disease and related dementias: focus on rivastigmine. *Curr Med Res Opin* 2002; **18**: 156–71.

36 Reading P, Luce A, McKeith I. Rivastigmine in the treatment of parkinsonian psychosis and cognitive impairment: preliminary findings from an open trial. *Mov Disord* 2001; **16**: 1171–4.

37 Finkel S. Effects of rivastigmine on behavioral and psychological symptoms of dementia in Alzheimer's disease. *Clin Ther* 2004; **26**: 980–90.

38 Liebel J. *Results of a 12-month post-marketing surveillance study with rivastigmine in patients with mild-to-moderately severe Alzheimer's disease. Pathways from Science to Effective Patient Management in Dementia: Novartis Satellite Meeting.* Istanbul, 2001.

39 Wilkinson D, Passmore A, Bullock R et al. A multinational, randomised, 12-week, comparative study of donepezil and rivastigmine in patients with mild to moderate Alzheimer's disease. *Int J Clin Pract* 2002; **56**: 441–6.

40 Sharma J. Cholinesterase inhibitors in Alzheimer's disease: donepezil or rivastigmine? *Int J Clin Pract* 2002; **56**: 414–15.

41 Gauthier S, Emre M, Farlow M et al. Strategies for continued successful treatment of Alzheimer's disease: switching cholinesterase inhibitors. *Curr Med Res Opin* 2004; **19**: 707–14.

42 Auriacombe S, Pere J, Loria-Kanza Y, Vellas B. Efficacy and safety of rivastigmine in patients with Alzheimer's disease who failed to benefit from treatment with donepezil. *Curr Med Res Opin* 2002; **18**: 129–38.

43 Skoog I, Lernfelt B, Landahl S et al. 15-year longitudinal study of blood pressure and dementia. *Lancet* 1996; **347**: 1141–5.

44 Kumar V, Anand R, Messina J, Hartman R, Veach J. An efficacy and safety analysis of Exelon in Alzheimer's disease patients with concurrent vascular risk factors. *Eur J Neurol* 2000; **7**: 159–69.

45 Erkinjuntti T, Skoog I, Lane R, Andrews C. Rivastigmine in patients with Alzheimer's disease and concurrent hypertension. *Int J Clin Pract* 2002; **56**: 791–6.

46 Erkinjuntti T, Skoog I, Lane R, Andrews C. Potential long-term effects of rivastigmine on disease progression may be linked to drug effects on vascular changes in Alzheimer brains. *Int J Clin Pract* 2003; **57**: 756–60.

47 Spencer C, Noble S. Rivastigmine. A review of its use in Alzheimer's disease. *Drugs Aging* 1998; **13**: 391–411.

48 Grossberg G. Cholinesterase inhibitors for the treatment of Alzheimer's disease: getting on and staying on. *Curr Ther Res Clin Exp* 2003; **64**: 216–35.

49 Inglis F. The tolerability and safety of cholinesterase inhibitors in the treatment of dementia. *Int J Clin Pract* 2002; **127**: 45–63.

50 Schmidt R, Lechner A, Petrovic K. Rivastigmine in outpatient services: experience of 114 neurologists in Austria. *Int J Clin Pract* 2002; **17**: 81–5.

51 Morganroth J, Graham S, Hartman R, Anand R. Electrocardiographic effects of rivastigmine. *J Clin Pharmacol* 2002; **42**: 558–68.

52 Grossberg G, Stahelin H, Messina J, Anand R, Veach J. Lack of adverse pharmacodynamic drug interactions with rivastigmine and twenty-two classes of medications. *Int J Geriatr Psychiatry* 2000; **15**: 242–7.

53 Verny M, Fremont P, Bourrin J. Reduced psychotropic drug use in patients with Alzheimer's disease receiving rivastigmine: results of the EXELAN study. *J Drug Assess* 2004; **7**: 123–32.

54 Suh D, Arcona S, Thomas S et al. Risk of antipsychotic drug use in patients with Alzheimer's disease treated with rivastigmine. *Drugs Aging* 2004; **21**: 395–403.

55 Souetre E, Thwaites R, Yeardley H. Economic impact of Alzheimer's disease in the United Kingdom. Cost of care and disease severity for non-institutionalised patients with Alzheimer's disease. *Br J Psychiatry* 1999; **174**: 51–5.

56 Hauber A, Gnanasakthy A, Snyder E et al. Potential savings in the cost of caring for Alzheimer's disease. Treatment with rivastigmine. *Pharmacoeconomics* 2000; **17**: 351–60.

57 Hauber A, Gnanasakthy A, Mauskopf J. Savings in the cost of caring for patients with Alzheimer's disease in Canada: an analysis of treatment with rivastigmine. *Clin Ther* 2000; **22**: 439–51.

58 Fenn P, Gray A. Estimating long-term cost savings from treatment of Alzheimer's disease. A modelling approach. *Pharmacoeconomics* 1999; **16**: 165–74.

59 Lamb H, Goa K. Rivastigmine. A pharmacoeconomic review of its use in Alzheimer's disease. *Pharmacoeconomics* 2001; **19**: 303–18.

60 Clegg A, Bryant J, Nicholson T et al. Clinical and cost-effectiveness of donepezil, rivastigmine, and galantamine for Alzheimer's disease. A systematic review. *Int J Technol Assess Health Care* 2002; **18**: 497–507.

61 Wolfson C, Oremus M, Shukla V et al. Donepezil and rivastigmine in the treatment of Alzheimer's disease: a best-evidence synthesis of the published data on their efficacy and cost-effectiveness. *Clin Ther* 2002; **24**: 862–86.

Acknowledgements

Figure 2 is adapted from Rosler *et al.*, 1999.[19]

Figure 3 is adapted from Farlow *et al.*, 2000.[25]

Figure 4 is adapted from Schneider *et al.*, 1998.[21]

Figure 5 is adapted from Kumar *et al.*, 2000.[44]

Figure 6 is adapted from Erkinjuntti *et al.*, 2003.[46]

Figure 7 is adapted from Spencer *et al.*, 1998.[47]

PATIENT NOTES
Dr Steve Illiffe

Treatment options for Alzheimer's disease – how do they work?

There are currently four symptom-controlling medicines available to treat people with Alzheimer's disease. Three of these drugs work in the earlier stages of the disease process (the acetylcholinesterase inhibitors – donepezil [Aricept®], galantamine [Reminyl®], rivastigmine [Exelon®)]), whilst one is available for when the disease has progressed further (memantine [Ebixa®]). The three medicines for early use slow down the clearance of vital transmitter chemicals, whilst the one used for more severe disease works partly by preventing the build up of toxic chemicals in, and between, brain cells. Acetylcholine is a transmitter chemical that is removed from the space between brain cells by cholinesterase – a regulator chemical (or 'enzyme') that 'cleans up' the cellular environment. If there is an alteration in the balance between acetylcholine and cholinesterase, then too little or too much communication between cells may occur. For example, normal levels of cholinesterase and a deficiency in acetylcholine results in reduced communication between the cells of the brain. Inhibiting cholinesterase activity using drugs such as donepezil, rivastigmine and galantamine, restores the balance between the two chemicals. Memantine works by stopping brain cells from accumulating calcium, which in large quantities is toxic to the cells; this over-accumulation of calcium is thought to be one aspect of the disease process that occurs in Alzheimer's disease.

Choosing which drug to use in early Alzheimer's disease depends upon the ease of its use, its associated benefits, together with any side-effects. Since the response to treatment varies significantly in different individuals, the dose of each drug needs to be carefully adjusted according to the patient's response and any emerging side-effects, and the drug switched to an alternative treatment where necessary.

Below, I have summarised the broad characteristics of the different drugs available to treat early Alzheimer's disease. The clinical and pharmacological evidence underpinning their use in practice is presented in detail in the chapters preceding this article.

Choosing which drug to use in early Alzheimer's disease depends upon the ease of its use, its associated benefits, together with any side-effects.

Particular patients may have a preference for one drug over another, and this should not be neglected.

The cholinesterase inhibitors

Donepezil has the advantage that it can be taken once a day, and appears to have fewer side-effects for the majority of people than the other two drugs in this class. It can help improve thinking, behaviour and performance of everyday tasks. These effects can persist for a year or, in some cases, longer.

Galantamine needs to be taken twice daily, and appears to have beneficial effects on thinking and also the behavioural symptoms of the disease. It does, however, have more side-effects than donepezil, particularly in the stomach and intestine, and cannot be taken safely with some other drugs, like the antibiotic erythromycin.

Rivastigmine must also be taken twice daily, and improves thinking, behaviour and performance of everyday tasks. There is some evidence that the effects can last for up to 5 years after starting treatment, though side-effects are more frequent than with donepezil. Rivastigmine may be particularly useful in reducing the occurrence of disturbed behaviour, and hallucinations or delusions.

However, the differences that I have highlighted between these three medicines are not so great that it is possible to say with certainty which is the best option, though this may change as experience of their use increases. In addition, particular patients (and their families and carers) may have a preference for one drug over another, and this should not be neglected.

Memantine

The last medication to think about is memantine, which is for moderate-to-severe stages of Alzheimer's disease. This drug has been shown to stabilise performance of everyday tasks, slows deterioration and maintains independence, at least for 6 months after starting treatment. Its side-effects appear to be similar to the other three drugs, despite the fact that it works in a different way. Like galantamine and rivastigmine, memantine also needs to be taken twice daily. Memantine is the most recent of the four medicines to be introduced in the UK, and as such we can expect more information about its benefits and drawbacks to emerge in the coming years. The benefits of memantine will probably be very different from those of the three early stage drugs, and will more likely be related to altered behaviour rather than improved thinking.

What can be expected from treatment?

Family members and friends of a person with early Alzheimer's disease who is taking any one of these treatments are an important source of information about their effectiveness for that individual. In particular, you should be looking out for whether the patient's memory and thinking have improved, and note down important examples where this appears to be the case. It is also important to observe how the individual lives from day-to-day, particularly if their mood stabilises, or they become more able to do ordinary but important things, from shopping and socialising to dressing and bathing. Again, the details matter, and they need to be reported to and discussed with the doctor, psychologist or nurse who is overseeing the treatment programme. This level of attention even allows goals for treatment to be made, and medicines tested against them.

It is important to observe how the individual lives from day-to-day, particularly if their mood stabilises, or they become more able to do ordinary but important things.

6. Improving practice

Dr Ian Greaves MBChB BDS BMsc MRCGP
General Practitioner, Gnosall, Stafford

Summary

<u>Dementia</u> is a debilitating condition which impacts greatly on patients and their families. Although the prevalence of dementia is increasing as a result of increased longevity and social demographic changes, most family physicians may only encounter one or two new cases annually. As a result, many GPs are unaware of how to diagnose and manage the condition effectively, despite being ideally placed within the patient community to identify early signs of the illness. Although these may be difficult to define, physicians should look for signs of deterioration of <u>cognitive</u> (short-term memory) and non-cognitive abilities (depression, delusions, behavioural changes) and difficulties in performing activities of daily living (dressing, shopping). The <u>acetylcholinesterase inhibitors</u> offer effective relief from the symptoms of dementia with the greatest benefit observed for those patients in whom treatment is initiated rapidly following formal diagnosis. Although the improvement following drug treatment can be dramatic, some patients continue to steadily deteriorate. Despite this, long-term data suggest that continued treatment may benefit all patients by improving quality of life and delaying nursing home placement. Patients and their carers should be well advised of the many support groups and facilities available within the community and should be kept fully informed as to the likely course of disease progression and treatment expectations.

☛ Remember that the author of the Improving Practice is addressing his healthcare professional colleagues rather than the 'lay' reader. This provides a fascinating insight into many of the challenges faced by doctors in the day-to-day practice of medicine (see Reader's Guide).

The challenge of dementia in primary care

Family physicians with an interest in dementia are few and far between. The Audit Commission in their *Forget Me Not* report of 2000 have shown that more than half of the GPs surveyed admitted that they did not know enough about dementia. Only 48% of those surveyed felt that they had received sufficient training to help them diagnose and manage

> More than half of GPs surveyed admitted that they did not know enough about <u>dementia</u>.

dementia effectively and only 54% recognised the importance of actively looking for early signs of <u>dementia</u>.

Negative attitudes persist amongst many family doctors with regard to the reporting of an early diagnosis of dementia, partly due to the distress that is evoked in patients and their families when they receive a positive diagnosis. However, a clear message needs to be communicated to family physicians: patients with dementia are interesting, challenging and rewarding to treat, and a proactive caring approach can greatly enhance their patient's and their family's or carer's quality of life.

The majority of patients diagnosed with dementia are managed in the community. It is therefore vitally important that this problem is seen as one that principally affects people who live in the community and who only rarely visit healthcare professionals for advice or management. As such, the primary healthcare team are probably best placed to identify patients with early signs of dementia.

Dementia has an enormous impact not only on the patient but also on their family and carers and society as a whole. Indeed the social pathology of dementia can dominate the management of these patients and can enhance or restrict their care plans. The stigma associated with dementia and its negative image as a <u>chronic</u> debilitating disease that has no cure with only very limited therapies has an enormous effect on both the public perception of the condition and the attitude of healthcare professionals.

Dementia is a syndrome with many causes. It may be easier to think of it as 'brain failure' in order to overcome some of the negative perceptions that exist amongst healthcare workers. Dementia then becomes comfortable and manageable rather than foreboding. Healthcare workers are used to dealing with patients who have heart failure and most family doctors feel comfortable with its diagnosis and management despite its multiple causes and poor prognosis.

There is also a significant misconception by a lot of community healthcare workers that dementia is only a problem where the patient has memory lapses. Given that the brain is an essential organ, failure of function produces dramatic effects beyond memory lapses.

Practical strategies in dementia care

Expressions of dementia

There are three main features that GPs should be aware of when establishing a diagnosis of dementia. These are outlined below.

Cognitive deficits

<u>Cognitive</u> expressions of dementia initially begin as a reduction in short-term memory, euphemistically referred to as 'senior moments'. Most people develop compensation mechanisms such as <u>confabulation</u>, social ritual or become grumpy. As such, it can be extremely difficult to spot early changes. There are also changes in the ability to perform and

interact socially. The reduction in verbal reasoning and loss of language skills can also result in social isolation.

Non-cognitive features

Non-cognitive features associated with dementia include depression, hallucinations, delusions, misidentifications and behavioural disturbances. Such features may be accompanied by agitation, aggression, wandering and sexual disinhibition, or these symptoms can occur independently. Behavioural changes with wandering, aggression and inappropriate behaviour usually herald a stage where coping at home becomes impossible, leading to a need for structured care in an appropriate setting.

Declining function

Further deterioration of brain function impacts on activities of daily living (ADLs), increasing the dependence of the patient upon others to look after them to survive. The patient presents with difficulties in feeding, dressing, toileting and activities such as using money, shopping or making telephone calls.

The burden of dementia in primary care

Most family physicians with a list of about 2000 patients will see about one or two new cases of dementia each year. As such, it is by no means a common condition. However, increased longevity and social demographic changes mean that dementia is going to become an increasing problem in the future. As a rule of thumb, the incidence of dementia doubles every 5 years in patients over 60 years: only 1% of the 60–64 year age group are affected, whereas dementia can be diagnosed in approximately 30% of all people aged 90 years.

Although its incidence is relatively low compared to say chest infections or cardiovascular disease, the problem of dementia represents an enormous drain on our resources and time. Several agencies are usually involved in the care programme and therefore the care plans set up to manage our patients demand good communication and multidisciplinary working practices.

> Although its incidence is relatively low compared to say chest infections or cardiovascular disease, the problem of dementia represents an enormous drain on our resources and time.

Dementia management

Early diagnosis of dementia is essential as there is a new range of drugs available that have been shown to have symptomatic benefit (in terms of cognition, behaviour and function) in this debilitating condition. These drugs seem to work better if we can introduce them at the earliest stage possible. Unfortunately the average time between suspicion of dementia and formal diagnosis can be several years.

Early diagnosis is also helpful in planning services for individuals including the initiation of other treatments for non-cognitive symptoms.

These interventions should include psychosocial approaches and maintenance of patients' independence by environmental manipulation. Social interaction can be improved with activity programmes and other interventions. It is important that a thorough assessment is also made to distinguish between dementia, depression and other confusional states. However, the differential diagnosis between dementia and other conditions is usually completed by secondary care services. The GP can help by checking the results of a full blood count and an erythrocyte sedimentation rate (ESR), a biochemical screen (including C-reactive protein, electrolytes, liver and thyroid function tests, vitamin B_{12} folate, VDRL, calcium and fasting blood glucose), an electrocardiogram (ECG) and midstream specimen of urine. Some authorities also recommend a chest X-ray. The results of these should be included in the referral letter.

The National Institute for Clinical Excellence (NICE) insists that only specialists should initiate acetylcholinesterase inhibitor treatment in patients with Alzheimer's disease. In contrast the Scottish Intercollegiate Guidelines Network (SIGN) encourages GPs to diagnose dementia and prescribe acetylcholinesterase inhibitors in straightforward cases. In addition, if GPs are to be involved in repeat prescribing, the guidance recommends they should do so only under an agreed shared care protocol with a clear end point. This means that monitoring and prescribing of acetylcholinesterase drugs in the community needs a carefully constructed integrated approach that uses group protocols and shared care arrangements. One of the milestones of the National Service Framework (NSF) for Older People is the production and implementation of shared care protocols for dementia. Most patients find access to secondary care more difficult than primary care and a more integrated service could therefore reduce the delay in diagnosis and thereby improve outcomes and compliance.

> Most patients find access to secondary care difficult and a more integrated service could therefore reduce the delay in diagnosis and thereby improve outcomes and compliance.

Although the labelling for the acetylcholinesterase inhibitors states that this class of drugs is indicated for symptomatic treatment there is a growing body of evidence to suggest that additional non-cholinergic actions may have additional benefits. Mild Alzheimer's disease is usually associated with a mini-mental state examination (MMSE) score of 21–26 and moderate disease with a score of between 10 and 20. Severe disease is considered to exist when the MMSE is below 10. Donepezil, rivastigmine and galantamine are all licensed for the treatment of mild-to-moderate Alzheimer's disease. In 2001, NICE recommended that treatment should not continue in patients in whom the MMSE has fallen below 12, although this guidance is due to be reviewed in 2005 (see Editor's note at the end of this article). However, withdrawal of these drugs can be problematic when we consider the expectations of a patient's family and carers. Such concerns can be minimised by the use of an explicit care plan that sets out the benchmarks of treatment interventions. It is best to avoid sudden changes and inform all individuals concerned of proposed changes in treatment.

Practical strategies for early diagnosis

Early diagnosis of <u>dementia</u> in routine care is difficult but not impossible. Firstly we need to get the message out to the community that early presentation helps. Obviously, the target population is the elderly. In our area we often go and talk at older people's clubs and social functions. If doctors cannot afford the time then there are plenty of volunteers in the Alzheimer's Society. The message needs to be upbeat and exciting to combat the negative image that prevails at present. We already do a lot of things well. For example, we can manage <u>cardiovascular</u> risk factors, encourage mental exercises, review medications to minimise the use of drugs with <u>cholinergic</u> side-effects and can treat concomitant conditions.

We can also use our position as family doctors to identify the early clinical signs of dementia. The elderly are seen much more often than other patients, and if doctors don't see them there are others in the primary healthcare team who do. The over 75s get seen by someone at least once a year. It's a case of having appropriate suspicion and knowing the patients well. What you are looking for is change. Remember some of the brighter people can exhibit a considerable change in their <u>cognitive</u> powers whilst others may have less of a change, but the fall off takes them below the coping level and becomes noticeable.

The advent of the new GP contract means we are now screening everyone for <u>cardiovascular disease</u>. Those at a high risk of arteriosclerosis are also at a high risk of <u>vascular</u> dementia. These high-risk patients regularly get examined and have bloods taken for <u>baseline renal</u> and lipid levels. They may even undergo an <u>electrocardiogram (ECG)</u>, as it is easy then to spot the difference when they have an <u>acute</u> event. This affords us an opportunity to add in a cognitive test to the cardiovascular assessment to spot changes when they do occur. Remember though that vascular dementia has a pattern of sudden decline and plateaus, whereas decline in Alzheimer's disease is gradual and progressive.

The Royal College of General Practitioners strongly recommend that GPs should be at the forefront of identifying dementia in older patients. In general they recommend that cognitive function be assessed in a systematic way. They recommend the following assessments, with a warning of cultural specificity:

- ask the patient the time to the nearest hour (orientation)
- give the patient an address to recall at the end of the test; the patient should repeat the address to ensure that it has been heard correctly (recall)
- ask the patient to count backwards from 20 to 1 (attention)
- ask the patient to draw the face of a clock with the fingers pointing at ten to eleven.

If the patient fails any of these initial assessments it is then necessary to move on to a full assessment.

> Remember some of the brighter people can exhibit a considerable change in their cognitive powers whilst others may have less of a change, but the fall off takes them below the coping level and becomes noticeable.

> The Royal College of General Practitioners recommend that GPs should be at the forefront of identifying <u>dementia</u> in older patients.

The facilities for looking after the elderly and especially those with dementia vary across the globe. In affluent countries the state offers both financial and physical help through the social services agencies. This can range from care plans designed to keep the patient at home through to some form of assisted, residential or nursing home accommodation.

In poorer countries the responsibility for care of the elderly falls entirely on the family. It is perceived as their responsibility to look after their relatives and this can cause an enormous strain. However, this model is fine as long as there are sufficient numbers of younger family members to support their elders.

Unfortunately, in richer countries the burden of eldercare is falling onto a smaller workforce, necessitating a greater role for the family in patients' care. This is borne out of the marked change in social demography as the population lives longer. Moreover, we have yet to experience the consequences of the post-war baby boomers reaching retirement age and the likely impact this will have on healthcare services.

Drug treatment

The rationale for early initiation of drug treatment is to delay the debilitating effects of this disease, improve quality of life for both patient and carer and to keep the patient in the community for longer. Inter-generational tensions arise as families struggle with the competing demands of a busy work life, childcare and eldercare. As a result there is a greater need for state provision often involving a complex series of care agencies. Therefore, not only are there sound clinical reasons for early intervention with appropriate drugs, but economic arguments also exist supporting such an approach.

The prescription and monitoring of drug treatment is an essential element of the care plan for dementia. The standardised MMSE for all its faults is still considered to be the best tool for this purpose. However, most clinicians feel that the MMSE alone does not give a good picture of the function of the patient and they therefore combine it with a good history taken from the patient's carer and an assessment of ADLs. The 'clock draw' test (discussed previously) is another good addition when monitoring a patient, and by comparing previous attempts of this task, it is an excellent visual assessment of disease progression.

The response to drug treatment can be dramatic, but some patients continue to deteriorate in a steady decline. Others show an initial response followed by deterioration below baseline.

Recent long-term data suggest that, as with many other conditions, there are continued benefits with continued treatment even if there is a decline in an individual's symptoms. We don't withdraw treatment when a patient's blood pressure starts to rise again or if diabetic control is lost. Even in the face of decline in dementia, continued treatment is associated with slower rate of decline, better quality of life and a delay to nursing home placement.

Patients treated with acetylcholinesterase inhibitors, for example, may experience a range of side-effects but common ones include

> The rationale for early initiation of drug treatment is to delay the debilitating effects of this disease and to keep the patient in the community for longer.

gastrointestinal symptoms of dyspepsia, nausea and vomiting and diarrhoea, and the central neurological symptoms of fatigue, insomnia and dizziness. Most patients tolerate these side-effects or can be managed with appropriate dose <u>titration</u>. In some cases treatment discontinuation or a switch to an alternative drug may be necessary. The GP is also ideally placed to take into account other medical conditions in which <u>cholinergic</u> stimulation may have an effect. Such effects are common in the elderly population and include <u>supraventricular cardiac conduction disorders</u>, asthma and <u>reversible airways disease</u>, bladder outflow disorders and seizures. Patients with these <u>comorbidities</u> should be reviewed more regularly and in more detail. The <u>renal</u> function of the patient should also be monitored, as patients with moderate renal impairment will require lower daily doses.

Donepezil can be given in a once-daily regimen and, as such, this may improve patients' compliance. The side-effect profile is dose related but the maximum dose is 10 mg. The dose range of rivastigmine is more complex and requires twice-daily dosing and a gradual titration. However, it has dual inhibitory effects on both <u>acetylcholinesterase</u> and <u>butyrylcholinesterase</u> in the brain. Unlike the other acetylcholinesterase inhibitors, rivastigmine has minimal potential for drug–<u>drug interactions</u>. Galantamine inhibits acetylcholinesterase and also modifies nicotinic cholinergic receptors. Thus, although all agents increase levels of <u>acetylcholine</u> in the brain, they also exhibit different individual non-cholinergic <u>pharmacology</u>.

Other services for patients with dementia

Drug treatments are only one arm of the therapeutic management of Alzheimer's disease. Any treatment plan should also include a comprehensive assessment of all the patients' and their carers' needs.

Admiral nurses (specialist <u>dementia</u> nurses, working in the community, with families, carers and supporters) and community-care teams that include mental health nurses, social workers and other support agencies offer carer support and it has been shown that timely intervention can prevent social breakdown. These teams can add focused and appropriate support required by patients' families.

Care plans should include the provision of respite and day-care services. The reduction in the financial viability of nursing homes has caused a lot of these facilities to close and has reduced the availability of good respite care. This is short sighted as the burden of care on the relatives rather than the severity of the dementia is often the determinant of permanent residential care admission.

The voluntary agencies are an invaluable resource in managing the care of dementia patients in the community. They provide a range of services from patient and carer education, support and advocacy through to befriending and sitting services. The voluntary workers frequently have a wealth of experience as they may have cared for their own relatives with dementia. Charitable societies such as the Alzheimer's Society provide a vast range of skilled and informed people to help with dementia.

> Admiral nurses and community-care teams offer carer support and it has been shown that timely intervention can prevent social breakdown.

Occupational therapists can assess the home of patients with dementia to provide aids and adaptations that manipulate the environment to help maintain independence. There has been an enormous amount of research that focuses on the abilities rather than the disabilities of people suffering from dementia. Dementia patients seem to do best in a friendly and familiar environment. Such things as the use of good lighting and primary colour decoration can be particularly beneficial. Familiar furniture contemporary with the time that the patient was at the peak of their performance has also been shown to be helpful.

Although communication through written and verbal language is reduced, patients with dementia can be stimulated with music and other art forms. The brain is a complex organ and there are many alternative ways of compensating for a reduced function. Such therapies certainly have a place in the rehabilitation of patients in the community.

The primary–secondary care interface

All patients who have been diagnosed with dementia in the community are referred to secondary care and, in the majority of cases, the service they get is excellent. It is very important that young patients with cognitive impairment (under 60 years of age) should be referred to secondary care as a matter of urgency as the likelihood of non-dementia pathology is far higher. Secondary-care services are not dissimilar to primary care in that they are stretched to breaking point. It is unfortunate that over a third of the family doctors in the UK surveyed in the *Forget Me Not* report felt that they did not have ready access to specialist advice. Specialist teams for older people with mental health problems were fully available in less than half of all areas and partly available in a further third. Additionally, the majority of secondary-care teams did not have a full complement of recommended core team members. NICE imposes a further burden on these services by recommending that only specialists initiate treatment with acetylcholinesterase inhibitors.

> Over a third of the family doctors in the UK surveyed in the *Forget Me Not* report felt that they did not have ready access to specialist advice.

The common sense approach to overcome these problems would seem to be to help each other. The 'carve out' model where a consultant assumes the care of a patient until they eventually die cannot be sustainable. Nor does the prevalence of the disease justify the transfer of memory clinics into primary care. Domiciliary visits increase costs and, whilst giving the consultant first hand experience of the social arrangements of the patient, may actually serve to lengthen waiting times. So the future of dementia care may be to come together to produce clearly defined pathways of care. This will serve to break down the tribal barriers of service provision, improve consistency and rapidity of diagnosis and set out best practice for management. This does not necessarily mean us doing anything different – just smarter.

In my own family practice the adult psychiatrists run the outpatient clinics at our surgery. This has reduced the stigma of the condition and brought the services closer to the patient. Moreover, the failures to attend have reduced from 30 to 1%. As family doctors we have gained in confidence in the diagnosis and treatment of a lot of other common psychiatric problems – it is amazing how much is diffused subconsciously into a doctor's brain over a cup of coffee with a consultant colleague. Similarly the background information we can offer to specialists is vital and is much better given verbally than in a three-page letter of referral. It is easy for us to help to prepare the patient for a consultant opinion both in the physical work-up with the blood tests and other things that need to be done. We can also use our position as the trusted family doctor to help them understand the process and guide them through the multidisciplinary assessments that lie in front of them. We already share resources – our practice nurses, community nurses, health visitors and their community psychiatric nurses (CPNs), elderly mentally infirm (EMI) beds, respite services, day hospitals and other therapeutic options.

Surely this is the best way forward for the elderly mentally ill. I am convinced we would use joined up thinking to agree mutual pathways of care with family doctors doing the things we are good at and get the best out of our consultant colleagues. It does not have to be as formal as outreach clinics. Perhaps we can agree to look at particular groups to get earlier identification of patients with suspected <u>dementia</u> and improve the quality of referral with all the basic investigations done. We can then monitor consultant-initiated therapies and enact treatment plans. We already do this for diabetics and for patients with <u>cardiovascular disease</u>. In turn the consultants would see our new referrals more quickly and bail us out if we phone them in a panic. However, Primary Care Trusts would have to acknowledge the effect of the change of prescribing on the drug budgets of GPs, given that the cost of treatment is approximately £800–1000 per patient per year.

Editor's note: This Improving Practice article by Dr Greaves first appeared in *Drugs in Context*, which was published in April 2004. As Dr Greaves highlights, guidance from the National Institute for Clinical Excellence (NICE) on the use of donepezil, galantamine, memantine and rivastigmine was undergoing review when this issue of *Drugs in Context* was published. However, as this edition of *BESTMEDICINE* goes to press (March 2005), the institute has issued preliminary guidance on the use of these drugs in the NHS, which reverses its original guidance and recommends against the use of these drugs for new patients. Whilst the institute acknowledges that each drug offers clinically relevant benefits, both in controlled clinical trials and in real clinical practice, it argues that economic evaluations puts these drugs outside the range of cost-effectiveness that NICE considers acceptable for the NHS. However, it is important to remember that this is preliminary guidance, and is subject to further consultation and review involving a number of parties, including patient support groups and the manufacturers of the drugs. Indeed, as we go to press, the opposition to this preliminary guidance has gathered pace, with the UK Health Minister, Stephen Ladyman, urging NICE to reconsider the wider implications of not approving the drugs' use, in particular the benefits and costs to carers as well as patients. Hundreds of people have also called for an end to dementia discrimination at a mass lobby of parliament organised by the Alzheimer's Society.

The final recommendation from NICE on the use of these drugs in Alzheimer's disease is not expected to be published until October 2005. In the intervening period, we will keep readers abreast of developments through our website (*www.bestmedicine.com*), and as soon as the final guidance from NICE is announced, we will publish a second edition of *BESTMEDICINE Alzheimer's Disease*, which will clarify what this guidance means for patients and their families. In the meantime, we hope that the information that you find in this book will be valuable when discussing long-term care with healthcare professionals.

Key points

- It is important that the primary healthcare team, as the first point of contact for many elderly patients, is able to recognise the early signs of dementia and instigate an effective programme of management.

- The deterioration of short-term memory and verbal reasoning, mood changes, behavioural abnormalities and difficulty performing activities of daily living all represent characteristic features of <u>dementia</u>.

- A proactive caring approach can greatly enhance patients' and caregivers' quality of life and can be both rewarding and interesting for the physician.

- Patients' families in particular may benefit from the level of specialist support offered by Admiral nurses and community care teams, which represent an invaluable resource in disease management.

- Addressing elderly audiences through social and community groups will increase the awareness of dementia and its early symptoms and may help to combat the negative image associated with mental illness.

- Early diagnosis can be aided by initiating a full blood count, a biochemical screen and a midstream specimen of urine, the results of which should be incorporated into the referral letter.

- Combining the MMSE with a clock-drawing exercise provides a more visual representation of disease progression.

- Drug treatment may dramatically slow disease progression in some patients whilst others may continue to deteriorate. Continued treatment may still benefit the patient, even if there is a decline in their symptoms.

- The discontinuation of drug treatment following a sudden deterioration in mental status, in line with current guidelines, should be fully explained in advance to the patient's family and carers.

PATIENT NOTES
Dr Steve Illiffe

The importance of the GP in managing Alzheimer's disease

The family doctor should be a source of help and support to the person with Alzheimer's disease and their family. He/she may suspect the disease at an early stage, but not feel certain enough to talk about it openly, so family members voicing concern can bring the subject into the open and allow a freer discussion. Doctors who have seen people in the last stages of the disease process may be afraid of it, and as such, may form inaccurate views of what Alzheimer's does to people in its early stages. They may not suspect Alzheimer's disease initially, but this does not mean that the possibility should not be discussed – on the contrary. And they may also attribute changes in thinking, behaviour and everyday activities to 'old age', which should be challenged.

The GP should know how important it is to get the views of family members, particularly if the individual affected believes that there is nothing wrong. At first the discussion may be in terms of 'memory problems', but as certainty and confidence grow it may be better to start to refer to Alzheimer's disease specifically. How and when to do this will depend on how the person affected responds to bad news, and here those who know them best must fill the gaps in the GP's knowledge. The GP should also be able to use and interpret a simple test of thinking and memory, and should also conduct simple blood tests that will rule out other causes of memory loss and muddled thinking, which include an under-active thyroid, vitamin B_{12} deficiency or undiscovered diabetes.

The GP should be able to distinguish between depression and dementia.

Working out whether someone really is developing early Alzheimer's disease can take time, but the GP should be able to distinguish between depression (which can also cause memory loss) and dementia, and should be very ready to refer the patient to an old-age psychiatrist for expert assessment. Effective use of medication depends not only on early recognition of Alzheimer's disease but also on early contact with specialists, because at the moment only they can start the treatments discussed in this edition of *BESTMEDICINE*. There is certainly no excuse for saying "nothing can be done".

There is certainly no 'rocket science' in any of this work, but there is careful detective work at the beginning, and continuity of care, empathy and practical assistance throughout.

The GP–specialist relationship

The family doctor can also share care with the specialist, by prescribing medication, checking for benefits and side-effects of medication, and by offering emotional support to the person with dementia and their carers on a regular basis. This gives the GP a chance to practice goal-oriented medicine, asking what the patient and their carers want out of possible treatment, and measuring the success of treatment against these personal goals. This will add to the assessments performed by specialists, whose employ standardised checklists and questionnaires that, whilst effective, may otherwise miss a crucial gain, like being able to go out for a drink with friends, or play with grandchildren. And the GP should also be able to point families towards sources of information and practical support, like the Alzheimer's Society and other voluntary groups in the locality, to achieve goals that the medical treatments cannot reach.

Continuing support for the patient and the family

This support from the GP needs to continue through the course of the disease, and should include advice on how to manage changing behaviour in moderate-to-severe dementia, and how to solve problems as they arise. Social services can provide practical help, and they can be contacted directly by the family, although information provided by the GP is important to help social workers understand both patients' and carers' needs. This involvement of the family doctor should continue even if the person with Alzheimer's disease needs to move into a care home, and should persist after the patient's death, as their family carries the memory of them and their illness with them. There is certainly no 'rocket science' in any of this work, but there is careful detective work at the beginning, and continuity of care, empathy and practical assistance throughout, all of which are vital for the well-being of the individual with Alzheimer's disease, and those around them.

Glossary

Aberrant motor – Abnormal movements.

Absorption – The movement and uptake of a drug into cells or across tissues (such as the skin, intestine and kidney).

Acetylcholine – A neurotransmitter widely used by nerve cells in both the peripheral and central nervous systems. The most abundant neurotransmitter in the peripheral nervous system.

Acetylcholinesterase – An enzyme that breaks down acetylcholine into its constituent products – acetate and choline.

Acetylcholinesterase inhibitors – Drugs (e.g. donepezil, galantamine, rivastigmine) that block the action of the acetylcholinesterase enzyme and thus increase levels of acetylcholine in the brain. Used therapeutically in the treatment of Alzheimer's disease.

Acute – A relatively short course of drug treatment lasting days or weeks rather than months. Also refers to the duration of a disease or condition.

ADAS-cog – The cognitive items in the Alzheimer's Disease Assessment Scale (ADAS) – a rating scale used to measure the severity of symptoms in Alzheimer's disease. The ADAS consists of 21 items, 11 of which measure cognitive function (ADAS-cog).

Adverse event – An unwanted reaction to a medical treatment.

Aetiology – The specific causes or origins of a disease, usually a result of both genetic and environmental factors.

Agonist activity – Mimicking or promoting the effects of another chemical (e.g. hormone or neurotransmitter) by stimulating the receptor or target site for that particular chemical.

Agonistic – Showing agonist activity.

Akathisia – The inability to sit still. Akathisia may occur as a side-effect of antipsychotic drugs, which are used to treat conditions including schizophrenia and bipolar disorder (alternatively called manic depression).

Alkalising gastric buffers – Substances that neutralise the acidic environment of the stomach, thus protecting the lining of the stomach from acid attack.

Allosteric activator – A substance that increases or decreases the activity of an enzyme by promoting the binding of a substrate (the substance on which an enzyme normally acts) to the enzyme.

Aminoadamantanes – Antagonists of N-methyl-D-aspartate (NMDA) glutamate receptors (e.g. memantine and amantadine) that have been shown to be effective in patients with Alzheimer's disease and Parkinson's disease.

Amyloid plaques – Abnormal deposits of the amyloid protein. The formation of amyloid plaques in the brain results in damage to nerve cells and may lead to Alzheimer's disease.

Anaesthesia – The loss of sensation and feelings of pain. Anaesthesia is induced in patients by the use of drugs to prevent pain and discomfort during surgery.

Anionic – Possessing a negative electrical charge.

Antioxidant – A substance that protects cell components from damage by oxidation. Examples of antioxidants include vitamins A, B1, B5, B6, C and E, and the minerals selenium and zinc.

Antispasmodic agents – Drugs that relax the smooth muscle in the walls of the intestine or bladder. Used to treat conditions in which the smooth muscle goes into spasms (e.g. irritable bowel syndrome).

Apoplectic – Caused by a stroke. Apoplexy is the sudden lack of oxygen to an area of the brain due to the rupture or blockage of a blood vessel.

Arteriosclerosis – Analagous to atherosclerosis. It is the deposition of fatty substances (mainly cholesterol) in the inner lining of an artery leading to the build-up of a substance known as an atheroma or plaque. This leads to hardening and narrowing of the arteries, and increases the risk of blood clots.

β-amyloid – A protein that forms thick deposits, or plaques, in the brains of patients with Alzheimer's disease.

β-amyloid precursor protein – The predecessor of β-amyloid.

β-amyloid polypeptides – Chains of β-amyloid protein.

Basal forebrain nuclei – Clusters of nerve cell nuclei in the base of the forebrain (the main mass of the brain). The cell nucleus is the structure within each cell that contains its genetic material.

Baseline – The starting point to which all subsequent measurements are compared. Used as a means of assessing improvement or deterioration during the course of a clinical trial.

Biomarkers – Biological substances or processes that act as indicators of disease. Used to measure the progress of a disease or the effects of treatment.

Blood–brain barrier – A physical obstacle that prevents certain substances from entering the brain. Essentially, it consists of the endothelial cells that line the capillaries supplying blood to the brain.

Blood serum – The clear, straw-coloured fluid component of blood after the clotting agents (e.g. fibrinogen and prothrombin) have been removed.

Brain atrophy – The shrinking or wasting away of brain tissue.

Bronchopneumonia – The most common form of pneumonia – the inflammation of the lungs due to infection. In bronchopneumonia, the inflammation is spread throughout the lungs in small patches.

Butyrylcholinesterase – An enzyme that breaks down the neurotransmitter acetylcholine. Butyrylcholinesterase is present in many tissues, including the brain and central nervous system and is also found in β-amyloid plaques as defined separately. The activity of butyrlycholinesterase is increased in the brains of people with Alzheimer's disease.

Calcium ions (Ca^{2+}) – Atoms of calcium that carry a double positive electrical charge due to the loss of two negatively charged electrons.

Carbamate – A chemical structure consisting of one nitrogen atom, one carbon atom, two oxygen atoms and one hydrogen atom.

Carbamylation – A chemical reaction between the amino group of a protein and cyanate derived from urea (a waste product of protein breakdown).

Cardiovascular disease – Disease of the heart and/or circulatory system. Stroke, coronary heart disease, atherosclerosis, hypertension, angina pectoris, cardiac arrhythmias and hypercholesterolaemia are all types of cardiovascular disease which represents the leading cause of death in the western world.

Cationic transport proteins – Proteins found in cell membranes that bind to substances with a positive charge (e.g. certain drugs and amino acids) and then transport these substances across the cell membrane.

Cerebral glucose metabolism – The production of energy through the breakdown of glucose, that enables the brain to function properly.

Cerebral hemisphere – One of the two halves of the cerebrum, the largest structure of the brain.

Cerebrospinal fluid (CSF) – A clear, colourless fluid that contains small quantities of glucose and protein. CSF fills the ventricles of the brain and nourishes and protects brain tissue.

Cerebrovascular – Pertaining to the blood vessels that supply blood to the brain.

Cholineacetyltransferase enzyme (ChAT) – An enzyme that catalyses the synthesis of acetylcholine in cholinergic nerve terminals.

Cholinergic – Pertaining to acetylcholine.

Cholinesterase inhibitors – see Acetylcholinesterase inhibitors.

Cholinomimetics – Agents that mimic the effects of the neurotransmitter acetylcholine by acting directly or indirectly on acetylcholine receptors.

Chronic – A prolonged course of drug treatment lasting months rather than weeks. Also refers to the duration of a disease or condition.

Co-administration – The simultaneous administration of more than one type of medication.

Co-agonist – A chemical that is required to allow the agonistic action of another chemical at its target receptor. For example, N-methyl-D-aspartate (NMDA)-receptors for the neurotransmitter glutamate also require the binding of the amino acid glycine before they become activated. In this case, glycine acts as a co-agonist to glutamate.

Cognitive – Pertaining to thought and mental processes.

Comorbid – A co-existing medical condition.

Confabulation – The fabrication of a story by someone to compensate for gaps in their memory. The person is not deliberately trying to deceive others but is simply trying to make sense of their past.

Contra-indication – Specific circumstances under which a drug should not be prescribed, for example, certain drugs should not be given simultaneously.

Cortex – The outer layer of certain organs, such as the brain, kidneys and adrenal glands.

Cortical neurones – Nerve cells in the cortex of the brain.

Cytochrome P450 (CYP) enzymes – A family of enzymes found in the liver that play an important role in the metabolism and detoxification of various compounds, including many drugs.

Dementia – A decline in mental ability, particularly intellectual functioning (or cognition). Dementia is usually caused by brain disease, is progressive (gradually gets worse) and is particularly common amongst the elderly.

Depolarisation – A reduction in the electrical charge that exists across muscle and nerve cell membranes when they are at rest. Normally, the interior of a nerve or muscle cell is electrically negative compared with the exterior because of the continual loss of positively charged sodium ions from inside the cell. Certain chemicals (e.g. neurotransmitters) reduce the electrical charge across the cell membrane by allowing sodium ions to flow into the cell. This is called depolarisation. If the cell is depolarised sufficiently, a nervous impulse is generated.

Divalent cations – An atom or group of atoms that carries a double positive electrical charge, gained by the loss of two negatively charged electrons. Calcium (Ca^{2+}) and magnesium (Mg^{2+}) ions are examples of divalent cations.

Dopamine – A chemical (neurotransmitter) in the brain that helps to transmit electrical impulses from one nerve cell to another. An imbalance in brain dopamine levels can cause brain dysfunction and disease, including schizophrenia and Parkinson's disease.

Dopaminergic agonists – Agents that activate dopamine receptors, thereby mimicking the effects of dopamine.

Double-blind – A clinical trial in which neither the doctor nor the patient are aware of the treatment allocation.

Drug interactions – In which the action of one drug interferes with that of another, with potentially hazardous consequences. Interactions are particularly common when the patient is taking more than one form of medication for the treatment of multiple disease states or conditions.

Dysphoria – An unpleasant mood: feeling dissatisfied, anxious, restless or sad.

Ecchymosis – Bruising.

Efficacy – The effectiveness of a drug against the disease or condition it was designed to treat.

Electrocardiogram (ECG) – A recording of the electrical activity of the heart. Useful for diagnosing disorders of the heart, many of which cause abnormal electrical patterns.

Electrolytic – Dissolving in water to form ions (electrically charged particles). These ions are able to conduct electricity. Examples of electrolytic substances are sodium and potassium salts. These dissolve in water to produce sodium (Na^+) and potassium (K^+) ions, respectively.

Elevated cholesterol – High levels of cholesterol in the blood. A major risk factor for coronary heart disease.

Endogenous ligand – A substance produced within the body which binds to a specific receptor.

Endpoint – A recognised stage in the disease process, used to compare the outcome in the different treatment arms of clinical trials. Endpoints can mark improvement or deterioration of the patient and signify the end of the trial.

Endothelial cells – Multifunctional cells that line blood vessels. Endothelial cells act as a barrier between the blood and other body tissues, attract white blood cells to the site of an infection, regulate blood flow and blood clotting, and control the contraction and relaxation of veins. The endothelial cells are collectively called the endothelium of a blood vessel.

Entorhinal cortex – An area of the brain that plays a major role in memory processes. The entorhinal cortex may be damaged in the early stages of Alzheimer's disease.

Enzymatic processes – Biochemical reactions in the body that are regulated by enzymes.

Enzyme – A protein produced by cells in the body that catalyses (increases the rate of) a specific biochemical reaction and is itself not destroyed in the process.

Epidemiology – The incidence or distribution of a disease within a population.

Episodic memory – The memory of events that an individual has experienced.

Erythrocytes – Red blood cells.

Esteratic – Capable of splitting ester bonds, the connections between a carbon atom and two oxygen atoms. Fats, such as cholesterol, are natural esters.

Excretion – The elimination of a drug or substance from the body as a waste product, for example, in the urine or faeces.

Extrapyramidal – Pertaining to a particular network of nerves in the brain. The extrapyramidal tract is involved in the control of skeletal muscle and hence movement. Damage to the nerves in the extrapyramidal system causes a disturbance in muscle tone and motor activity.

Extrapyramidal symptoms (EPS) – Symptoms caused by damage to or degeneration of the extrapyramidal tract. EPS commonly includes involuntary movements, tremors, rigidity, restlessness and changes in breathing and heart rate. EPS occur as a side-effect of some antipsychotic drugs.

Familial – Inherited.

Fasting blood glucose test – Measurement of the amount of sugar (glucose) in the blood after the person has not eaten for at least 6 hours. The test can be used to show whether a person has diabetes.

Focal neurological signs – Signs of damage to a particular area of the brain. For example, damage to the frontal lobe may cause dementia and epilepsy, whilst damage to the parietal lobe causes a disturbance in sensation.

Free radicals – Atoms or molecules that contain an unpaired electron and are highly reactive at cellular structures, because they take electrons from other molecules to become more stable. This process, known as oxidation, is toxic to many cells and can result in cellular damage. Free radicals are the by-products of both normal and pathological processes within the body.

Frontal lobes – The front surface of the left and right cerebral hemispheres of the brain. Important in the voluntary control of movement, behaviour and aspects of personality.

Fronto–temporal – Pertaining to the frontal and temporal lobes of the brain.

G1 isoform – One version of a particular protein. Some proteins exist in more than one form. The different forms, or isoforms, have the same function but are slightly different from each other, possibly in terms of their structure.

Genetic predisposition – An individual's susceptibility to developing a disease or condition as a result of their genetic make-up.

Genotype – The genetic information carried by each individual that acts as a 'blueprint' for that individual.

Glial cells – Cells in the brain that surround the nerve cells, providing support, protection and nourishment. They also help to maintain the correct balance of ions in the brain and produce the fatty coating of neurones.

Glutamate – An excitatory amino acid neurotransmitter found in the brain and spinal cord. Glutamate is involved in learning and memory, and under certain conditions (including Alzheimer's disease) it can cause nerve cell death.

Glycated – A molecule having undergone the attachment of additional glucose molecules. Such reactions commonly occur between proteins and hexose sugars, leading to the formation of glycated proteins. An example of one such protein is haemoglobin (the pigment in red blood cells). This reacts with glucose to form glycated haemoglobin.

Glycine – An inhibitory amino acid neurotransmitter found in the brain and spinal cord. Glycine is the simplest of the amino acids.

Hemiparesis – Muscular weakness or paralysis on one side of the body only.

Hepatic – Pertaining to the liver.

Hepatotoxicity – Being toxic to the liver; causing liver damage.

Higher cortical – Pertaining to the parts of the cerebral cortex (the outer surface of the main bulk of the brain) where the most complicated thought processes occur. Nerve cells in the cerebral cortex are arranged into six layers and the processing of information is hierarchical. Thus, complicated thought processes, such as decision-making and the planning of movements, take place in the higher layers.

Hippocampus – An area of the brain that plays an important role in learning and the storage of long-term memories. It is located in the temporal lobe, which is itself located to the side of the cerebral hemispheres. The hippocampus is often used experimentally to study synaptic plasticity and long-term potentiation (LTP).

Hydrocephalus – A reversible brain disorder caused by the accumulation of cerebrospinal fluid (CSF) in the ventricles of the brain, leading to enlargement of the ventric and, consequently, the compression of brain tissue. The condition may lead to the loss of any functions controlled by the area of compressed brain tissue. Dementia, difficulty walking and urinary incontinence are all symptoms of hydrocephalus.

Hypercalcaemia – Abnormally high levels of calcium in the blood. Possible causes of hypercalcaemia include cancer, the overproduction of parathyroid hormone (which helps to regulate blood calcium levels) and excessive intake of vitamin D. Hypercalcaemia causes nausea, vomiting, lethargy, depression, thirst and excessive urination. If left untreated, it may lead to an irregular heartbeat, kidney failure, coma and ultimately death.

Hyperphosphorylated – Having had multiple phosphate groups (one phosphorus atom and four oxygen atoms) added.

Hyperphosphorylation – The addition of multiple phosphate groups to a molecule, such as a protein.

Hypertension – Excessively high blood pressure.

Hypocholinergic – A lack or deficiency of the neurotransmitter acetylcholine; a common feature in the brains of patients with Alzheimer's disease.

Hyperthyroidism – The overproduction of thyroid hormones by the thyroid gland, which leads to over-activity of the body's metabolism, resulting in hyperactivity, insomnia, anxiety, increased appetite, diarrhoea and weight loss.

Ideation – The process of forming ideas in the mind.

Intracellular – Within a cell.

Intracerebroventricular – Within the ventricles of the brain. These are four cavities within the brain that are linked by a series of ducts. The ventricles are filled with cerebrospinal fluid, which helps to nourish and protect the brain.

In vivo – Used with reference to experiments performed within the living cell or organism.

In vitro – 'In glass'. Used with reference to experiments performed outside the living system in a laboratory setting.

Kinetics – The rate at which a chemical reaction occurs.

Lateral ventricles – Two of the four fluid-filled cavities in the brain. The ventricles are filled with cerebrospinal fluid which helps to nourish and protect the brain. The lateral ventricles are the two largest ventricles.

L-dopa (levodopa) – A drug used to treat Parkinson's disease. Unlike many drugs, L-dopa penetrates the blood–brain barrier (the endothelial cells that line the capillaries supplying blood to the brain and stop many substances from entering the brain). Once in the brain, L-dopa is converted into the neurotransmitter, dopamine, thereby helping to restore the deficit in brain dopamine levels that characterises Parkinson's disease.

Lewy body – An abnormal aggregate of protein (α-synuclein) inside a nerve cell that is commonly associated with Parkinson's disease, Lewy body dementia and other neurodegenerative disorders.

Ligand-gated ion channel – A protein channel in a cell membrane that opens or closes in response to the binding of a specific molecule (ligand), allowing the flow of ions (electrically charged atoms) into or out of the cell. The nicotinic acetylcholine receptor is an example of a ligand-gated ion channel.

Long-term potentiation (LTP) – An increase in the strength of synaptic transmission between two nerve cells following the repetitive use of the synapse. A form of synaptic plasticity that is thought to form the basis of learning and memory storage.

Macrocytic anaemia – A form of anaemia characterised by abnormally large red blood cells. The blood is unable to carry sufficient oxygen to the body's organs, resulting in tiredness, shortness of breath and pale skin. A deficiency of folic acid is one possible cause of macrocytic anaemia.

Magnesium ions (Mg^{2+}) – Atoms of magnesium that carry a double positive electrical charge due to the loss of two negatively charged electrons.

Magnetic resonance imaging (MRI) – An imaging technique that uses the influence of a large magnet to polarise hydrogen atoms within living tissues and produce a picture of the body's internal organs and structures that is far superior to that obtained using X-rays. MRI is used to diagnose a number of conditions, including cancer, cardiovascular disease, and disorders of the bones, joints or muscles.

Malaise – A vague feeling of illness or discomfort.

Malonate – A chemical that is toxic to mitochondria.

Markov model – A statistical model that is commonly used to analyse systems that may exist in different states, such as the human face. The model measures the probability of the system being in a given state at a given time point, the amount of time the system spends in a given state and the expected number of transitions between different states.

Mechanism of action – The manner in which a drug exerts its therapeutic effects.

Medial septum – An area of the brain that plays a major role in memory formation and storage. Damage to this part of the brain can cause memory loss (amnesia). The medial septum contains a high proportion of cholinergic neurones.

Meta-analysis – A set of statistical procedures designed to amalgamate the results from a number of different clinical studies. Meta-analyses provide a more accurate representation of a particular clinical situation than is provided by individual clinical studies.

Metabolism – The process by which a drug is broken down within the body.

Metabolites – The products of metabolism.

Microglia – Cells in the brain that digest and destroy foreign substances. Sometimes known as brain macrophages. Microglia are normally inactive, and are only activated when stimulated by an antigen (a foreign substance that triggers an immune response).

Microsomal enzyme – An enzyme found in microsomes, the small vesicles in cells in which proteins are synthesised.

Microtubule protein – Proteins that make up microtubules, such as tubulin and tau protein. Microtubules are minute, hollow, cylindrical tubes present in most animal cells. They provide structural support for cells and help to transport materials within cells.

Mitochondria – The energy-producing units of the body's cells (singular: mitochondrion). They are small, spherical or rod-shaped structures that are enclosed by a double membrane. The outer membrane is smooth, while the inner membrane is highly folded to form finger-like projections.

Moiety – A segment of a molecule.

Monomeric – Having the property of a monomer – a simple molecule that can combine with identical or similar molecules to form long molecular chains (polymers).

Monotherapy – Treatment with a single drug.

Monovalent cations – An atom or group of atoms that carries a single positive electrical charge. They gain the positive charge by losing negatively charged electrons, in this case one electron (hence the single positive charge). Examples of monovalent cations include sodium (Na^+) and potassium (K^+) ions.

Morbidity – A diseased condition or state or the incidence of a disease within a population.

Mortality – The death rate of a population. The ratio of the total number of deaths to the total population.

Motor incoordination – Clumsy or awkward movement. Poor handwriting, problems with balance, poor sports ability and pronounced delays in developmental motor milestones (e.g. sitting, crawling and walking) are all possible symptoms of motor incoordination.

Multicentre – A clinical trial conducted across a number of treatment centres, either abroad or in the same country.

Multifactorial – A disease or state arising from more than one causative element.

Muscarinic – Pertaining to the neurotransmitter acetylcholine. Describes a substance that produces or mediates the effects of acetylcholine.

Muscarinic receptor – A receptor that responds to acetylcholine and related compounds, including the mushroom poison, muscarine. Located on smooth muscle, cardiac muscle, some nerve cells in the central nervous system (CNS) and glands.

Myocardial infarction (MI) – Commonly known as a heart attack, MI is defined as permanent damage to an area of heart muscle caused by a lack of blood supply and hence an inadequate supply of oxygen. The most common cause is a blood clot that blocks the coronary arteries. The characteristic symptoms of a heart attack are a crushing pain in the chest that radiates into the shoulders or arms. One out of every five deaths is due to a heart attack.

N-demethylation – A chemical reaction involving the removal of a methyl group from the N-terminal (the end of the molecule containing a nitrogen atom) of the molecule or compound in question.

Neocortex – The outer surface of the cerebral hemispheres, which form the main bulk of the brain. The neocortex is the most advanced part of the brain and is responsible for more complex thought processes, such as learning, language and memory.

Neurodegenerative – Characterised by the deterioration of the central nervous system (CNS) and loss of nerve cells.

Neurofibrillary tangles – Knots of twisted tau protein fibres commonly found in the nerve cells of people with Alzheimer's disease. Tau protein normally assists in the formation of microtubules, which are hollow tubes that help to support cells and transport nutrients within them. In Alzheimer's disease, however, the tau protein is abnormal and the microtubules collapse.

Neurohormone – A hormone involved in the functioning of the nervous system.

Neuronal cytoskeleton – The network of protein filaments within nerve cells that helps them to maintain their shape.

Neuronal sprouting – The growth of new protrusions from nerve cells.

Neurones – Nerve cells. Neurones transmit electrical impulses (nerve impulses) throughout the nervous system. The nervous system contains billions of neurones.

Neuropsychiatric Inventory (NPI) scale – A questionnaire used to determine the extent of disturbed behaviour in patients with dementia. It also provides an indication of the distress experienced by the patient's carer as a result of the disturbed behaviour. The questionnaire is completed by the patient's physician in collaboration with the patient's carer. It covers 12 areas of disturbed behaviour, including delusions, hallucinations, anxiety, irritability and eating disturbances.

Neurosyphilis – Syphilitic infection of the brain or spinal cord that may ultimately result in dementia. Neurosyphilis can also cause muscle weakness in the limbs, which can eventually turn into total limb paralysis. Infection of the spinal cord can cause uncoordinated leg movements, urinary incontinence and pain in the limbs and abdomen.

Neurotransmitter – A chemical in the nervous system that transmits nervous impulses from one nerve cell to another across the junctions (synapses) between cells. Examples include acetylcholine, noradrenaline, serotonin and dopamine.

Niacin – One of the B group of vitamins, niacin is essential for the normal functioning of the nervous system and the gastrointestinal tract, being involved in the synthesis of a number of enzymes. It also acts to reduce blood cholesterol levels.

Niacin deficiency – Insufficient niacin in the body.

Nicotinic receptors – A family of proteins on the surface of muscle cells and neurones that respond to nicotine and acetylcholine and mediate the biological effects of these two chemicals. The other type of acetylcholine receptor is the muscarinic receptor. Nicotinic and muscarinic receptors are collectively called cholinergic receptors.

Noradrenaline – A monoamine neurotransmitter. It is also a hormone produced by the adrenal glands that stimulates the sympathetic nervous system. This results in an increased heart rate, the release of energy from fat and the release of glucose from the liver.

Noradrenaline release – The release of noradrenaline from nerve endings or the adrenal glands.

Normal pressure hydrocephalus – See Hydrocephalus.

Nucleus Basalis Magnocellularis (NBM) – Also known as the Nucleus Basalis of Meynert, it is part of the brain involved in learning and memory. Located towards the base of the brain in the forebrain. Cholinergic neurones from the NBM pass into many areas of the cerebral cortex (the outer layer of the brain), and are amongst the first neurones to die in Alzheimer's disease.

Nucleus Basalis of Meynert (NBM) – See Nucleus Basalis Magnocellularis.

Oestrogens – Sex hormones that are mainly produced in the ovaries of women. In men, oestrogens are produced in small amounts by the adrenal glands. Oestrogens are essential for the normal development and functioning of the female reproductive system.

Open-label – A clinical trial in which all participants (i.e. the doctor and the patient) are aware of the treatment allocation.

Ovariectomised – Having had the ovaries removed.

Oxidation – A chemical process involving either the removal of electrons from an atom or atoms within a molecule, the removal of a hydrogen atom from a molecule or the addition of an oxygen atom to a molecule. Oxidation can lead to the production of free radicals, which cause damage to cell components, such as proteins and DNA.

Oxidative – Pertaining to oxidation.

P300 latency – A measure of cognitive function. It involves measuring the speed of the brain's response to a sudden sound using an electroencephalographic (EEG) system to record the electrical activity of the brain. A delay in the appearance of sound-provoked brain waves is an indication of memory impairment. The test is used in the diagnosis of dementia.

p-value – In statistical analysis, a measure of the probability that a given result occurred by chance. If the p-value is less than or equal to 0.05 then the result is usually considered to be statistically significant, and not due to chance.

Parietal lobe – An area of the brain located towards the back of the cerebral hemispheres, which is involved in the processing of sensations.

Passive avoidance response – A behavioural test in rodents that is used to screen drugs that affect memory and learning. Rodents are trained to avoid punishment (e.g. an electric shock) by avoiding certain behaviours (e.g. exploring). The animals are re-tested after receiving a particular drug to see whether they have retained the avoidance behaviour.

Pathobiology – The biology of a particular disease.

Pathogenesis – The processes involved in the development of a particular disease.

Pathophysiology – The functional changes that accompany a particular syndrome or disease.

Peripheral nervous system – The division of the nervous system that provides a means of communication between the central nervous system (CNS) and the organs of the body.

Peripherally mediated salivation – Stimulation of the production of saliva via neurones in the peripheral nervous system.

Pharmacodynamics – The physiological and biological effects of a drug, including its mechanism of action.

Pharmacokinetics – The activity of the drug within the body over a period of time.

Pharmacology – The branch of science that deals with the origin, nature, chemistry, effects and uses of drugs.

Phosphotau protein – The phosphorylated form of tau protein. Phosphorylated means having had a phosphate group added. Phosphotau protein is found in high concentrations in the cerebrospinal fluid of patients with Alzheimer's disease.

Pick's disease – A form of dementia caused by the degeneration of the frontal and temporal lobes of the brain, leading to a loss of intellect and the inability to speak or understand words.

Piperidine – A biologically active chemical found in pepper and cannabis. Forms part of the structure of many antipsychotic drugs.

Placebo – An inert substance with no specific pharmacological activity.

Placebo-controlled – A clinical trial in which a proportion of patients are given placebo in place of the active drug.

Plasma protein binding – The binding of substances that circulate in the blood (e.g. a drug or hormone) to proteins present in the fluid component of blood (plasma), such as albumin.

Plateau of inhibition – The levelling off of the inhibitory effect of a compound at a certain concentration.

Pooled analysis – The amalgamation and processing of data derived from multiple clinical trials.

Positron emission tomography (PET) – An imaging technique that uses radioactive substances to visualise and measure the metabolic and physiological functioning of particular structures within the body (e.g. heart, brain). A radioactive substance is injected into, or inhaled by, the patient. The radiation emitted is detected and converted into colour-coded images, providing a three-dimensional image of the structure under investigation.

Postsynaptic – Occurring after a synapse; the junction of two nerve cells.

Postsynaptic receptors – Proteins located on the postsynaptic membrane of a nerve cell that have particular affinity for a certain neurotransmitter. The receptors 'receive' information transmitted from the previous nerve cell and mediate the biological effects of a particular neurotransmitter.

Potentiating effect – Making something more effective or more active.

Presenilin 1 and 2 – Two proteins that form part of an enzyme complex responsible for the formation of β-amyloid peptide from β-amyloid precursor protein.

Presynaptic – Occurring before a synapse; the junction between two nerve cells.

***Proteus* bacteria** – A group of small, rod-shaped bacteria that are mainly found in soil, where they help to break down organic matter. In humans, they are a common cause of urinary tract infections.

Pseudo-irreversible inhibitor – A drug, the inhibitory effects of which persist for much longer than it resides in the plasma (e.g. rivastigmine).

Psychotropic – Affecting the mind and mental processes.

Pulmonary – Pertaining to the lungs.

Pulmonary artery – Carries deoxygenated blood from the right ventricle of the heart to the lungs, where it is oxygenated.

Pulmonary embolism – Blockade of the pulmonary artery by a blood clot. This causes shortness of breath, difficulty in breathing and, if left untreated, death.

Rapid Eye Movement (REM) density – The number of rapid eye movements per unit of time during REM sleep (the period of sleep when a person dreams).

Rater-blinded – Pertaining to the design of a clinical trial whereby the investigator evaluating the patient's response to the test treatment is unaware of which treatment the patient has received.

REM latency – The time from when a person first falls asleep to the first occurrence of REM sleep (the period of sleep when a person dreams).

Renal – Pertaining to the kidneys.

Renal tubular acidosis (RTA) – The inability of the kidneys to excrete the acid produced by the body. Consequently, the blood becomes more acidic than normal and the urine less acidic. RTA may lead to softening of the bones, the development of kidney stones and abnormally low blood potassium levels (causing tiredness and muscle weakness).

Reversible airways disease – Diseases of the pulmonary system (e.g. asthma), in which airflow is temporarily obstructed by the narrowing or inflammation of the airways. Reversible with appropriate treatment.

Rhinitis – Inflammation of the mucous membrane lining the nose. Symptoms include sneezing, a runny, itchy nose, and nasal congestion (blocked nose). Rhinitis is commonly caused by an allergy to an airborne substance, such as pollen or dust. Hay fever is rhinitis caused by an allergy to grass pollen.

Safety and tolerability – The side-effects associated with a particular drug and the likelihood that patients will tolerate a drug treatment regimen.

Selective serotonin reuptake inhibitor (SSRI) – A drug that prevents the reuptake of serotonin by nerve terminals in the central nervous system, thereby increasing serotonin levels in the brain. Such drugs are commonly used to treat depression and examples include fluoxetine (Prozac®), paroxetine (Seroxat®) and sertraline (Lustral®).

Serotonin – A neurotransmitter in the brain that plays an important role in the regulation of mood, sexuality and food intake.

Serotonin reuptake inhibitor – See Selective serotonin reuptake inhibitor (SSRI).

Serum – The clear, straw-coloured fluid component of blood, after the clotting agents (e.g. fibrinogen and prothrombin) have been removed.

Serum calcium test – A procedure that measures the amount of calcium in the fluid portion of blood. This test is usually performed to screen for diseases of the kidneys or parathyroid glands.

Single-blind – A clinical trial in which only the patient is unaware of the treatment allocation.

Single Photon Emission Computed Tomography (SPECT) – A computerised imaging technique that uses gamma rays (a form of electromagnetic radiation) to produce a series of images or 'slices' through a patient's body. The patient is first injected with a substance that emits gamma rays. Images of the patient are then taken from different angles using a camera that detects gamma rays.

Socioeconomic impact – Social and economic factors that characterise the influence of a disease. Incorporates the financial cost incurred by the healthcare provider, the patient and the wider economy.

Soluble β-amyloid precursor protein release – Release of the soluble fragment of β-amyloid precursor protein from nerve cells.

Somatic – Pertaining to the physical body as opposed to the mind or pertaining to the part of the nervous system that controls voluntary functions.

Somnolence – Drowsiness or sleepiness.

Spasticity – Increased rigidity of muscles, leading to stiffness and restricted movement. Can be accompanied by paralysis.

Spatial memory – The recollection of how items are organised spatially within one's immediate environment (e.g. in a room).

Sporadic – Occurring irregularly; having no pattern or order.

Statistical significance – A measure of the probability that a given result derived from a clinical trial – be it an improvement or a decline in the health of the patient – is due to a specific effect of drug treatment, rather than a chance occurrence.

Steady-state – A condition whereby all the components of a system remain at a constant concentration and do not fluctuate. For example, the steady-state concentration of a drug in the blood is the concentration at which drug levels are constant.

Stepwise deterioration – Deterioration that occurs in recognised stages.

Striatal axial slices – Slices of tissue taken from the striatum of the brain *post mortem* in an axial plane. That is, running from the front to the back of the body. Also known as a transverse section.

Striatal lesions – Injury or damage to the nerve cells of the striatum.

Striatum – Part of the extrapyramidal motor system of the brain that has a striped or striated appearance. The striatum is involved in the control of movement, balance and walking and may be damaged in patients with Parkinson's disease. The nerve cells of the striatum require dopamine to function.

Subclinical ischaemia – Ischaemia (reduced blood supply) that is not severe enough to cause obvious signs or symptoms.

Subdural haematoma – A blood clot situated in the space between the middle and outer meninges (the membranes that surround and protect the brain and spinal cord). The most common cause of a subdural haematoma is a blow to the head. As the collection of clotted blood enlarges, it presses against the brain tissue causing headaches, confusion, drowsiness and weakness or paralysis on one side of the body.

Succinylcholine-type – Resembling succinylcholine, a compound consisting of two molecules of acetycholine linked together. It imitates the actions of acetylcholine but is degraded by the enzyme pseudocholinesterase rather than acetylcholinesterase. Used as a short-term muscle relaxant. Also known as suxamethonium chloride or scoline.

Sulphate conjugation – A biochemical reaction that occurs in the liver to deactivate many drugs. It involves the attachment of a sulphate group (one atom of sulphur and four atoms of oxygen) to the drug. This changes the structure of the drug, which is then excreted via the kidneys.

Supraventricular cardiac conduction disorders – The irregular conduction of the electrical impulse that precedes a heartbeat in the atria (upper chambers of the heart).

Surrogate markers – Laboratory or physical parameters that are used as a substitute for a direct biological measurement, such as how a patient feels, or how effective a particular treatment is.

Synapse – A junction between two nerve cells where the electrical activity in one nerve cell influences the excitability of the other.

Synaptic cleft – The space separating two nerve cells at a synapse. Neurotransmitters are released from the ends of nerve cells into the synaptic cleft in small vesicles (membrane-bound sacs). The vesicles travel across the synaptic cleft to the next nerve cell, where the neurotransmitter changes the electrical charge across the nerve cell membrane, leading to a nervous impulse. In this way, nerve impulses are transmitted from one nerve cell to another.

Synaptic noise – Random fluctuations in nerve cell membrane potential (the electrical charge across the membrane) at the synapse. Generally insufficient to cause the transmission of an electrical impulse between the two nerve cells.

Synaptic plasticity – An increase in the strength of synaptic transmission between two nerve cells following the repetitive use of the synapse. Thought to form the basis of learning and memory storage. Long-term potentiation (LTP) is a form of synaptic plasticity.

Syncope – Fainting, due to insufficient blood supply to the brain.

Systemic half-life – The time taken for half the amount of a drug to be removed from the bloodstream.

Tau protein – A protein that together with tubulin, forms the basis of microtubules – hollow cylindrical tubes present within most cells that provide the cell with structural support. In Alzheimer's disease, however, tau protein is abnormal and the microtubules collapse.

Temporal lobe – An area of the brain located to the side of the cerebral hemisphere. Important in the processing of auditory information and language.

Tertiary alkaloid – A class of organic compounds containing a nitrogen atom connected to three (hence the term tertiary) carbon-based groups of atoms. Alkaloids occur naturally in plants and tend to be biologically active in humans (e.g. morphine, nicotine, cocaine).

Tetrameric enzyme – An enzyme consisting of four subunits linked together.

Titrated – Having undergone titration. Dose titration describes the determination of the lowest dose of a particular drug that will give the desired effect with the minimum of side-effects.

Upregulation – An increase in the number of target receptors for a given chemical on the cell surface. This leads to an increase in the response that normally occurs when the relevant chemical binds to the receptor.

Vascular – Pertaining to the blood vessels.

Vitamin B$_{12}$ deficiency – Insufficient vitamin B$_{12}$ within the body. B vitamins are necessary for the formation of red blood cells, the repair of cells and tissues and the synthesis of DNA. A deficiency in vitamin B$_{12}$ results in nerve damage, causing tingling and numbness in the hands and feet, and mental changes, such as confusion, irritability and depression.

Voltage dependent – Being dependent on the voltage potential across a cell membrane (also known as the membrane potential) – the difference between the electrical charge inside the cell and that on the outside of the cell.

Wash-out period – A period of time in a clinical trial during which patients do not receive any treatment so that the effects of previous treatments are allowed to wear off.

Wechsler Adult Intelligence – A measure of intelligence using the Wechsler Adult Intelligence Scale (WAIS). The WAIS test consists of 11 subtests, six of which are verbal tests and five of which are performance tests. WAIS was developed for use in clinical, educational and research settings.

Useful contacts

The organisations listed below represent an accurate cross-section of what we believe to be reliable and up-to-date sources of information on Alzheimer's disease and its management.

The Alzheimer's Society

Gordon House
10 Greencoat Place
London
SW1P 1PH
Email: *enquiries@alzheimers.org.uk*
Helpline: 0845 300 0336
Website: *http://www.alzheimers.org.uk/*
Registered charity

Alzheimer Scotland

22 Drumsheugh Gardens
Edinburgh
EH3 7RN
Email: *alzheimer@alzscot.org*
Helpline: 0808 808 3000
Website: *http://www.alzscot.org*
Registered charity

Alzheimer's Disease International

64 Great Suffolk Street
London
SE1 0BL
Email: *info@alz.co.uk*
Tel: 020 7981 0880
Website: *http://www.alz.co.uk/*
Registered charity

Age Concern

Astral House
1268 London Road
London
SW16 4ER
Email: *ace@ace.org.uk*
Information line: 0800 00 99 66
Website: *http://www.ageconcern.org.uk/*
Registered charity

Carers UK

20–25 Glasshouse Yard
London
EC1A 4JT
Email: *info@carersuk.org*
Carers line: 0808 808 7777
Tel: 020 7490 8818
Website: *http://www.carersonline.org.uk*
Registered charity

Alzheimer's Research Trust

Livanos House
Granhams Road
Cambridge
CB2 5LQ
Email: *enquiries@alzheimers-research.org.uk*
Tel: 01223 843899
Website: *http://www.alzheimers-research.org.uk/*
Registered charity

Dementia Relief Trust

6 Camden High Street
London
NW1 0JH
Email: *info@fordementia.org.uk*
Tel: 020 7874 7210
Website: *http://www.dementiarelief.org.uk*
Registered charity

Best Treatments UK

Website:
http://www.besttreatments.co.uk/btuk/home.html
Produced by the British Medical Association

NHS Direct

Website: *http://www.nhsdirect.nhs.uk/*

Index

Notes

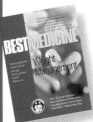
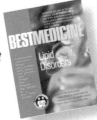
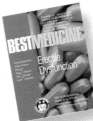
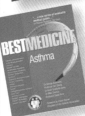
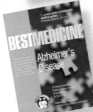
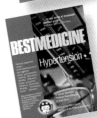
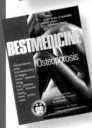
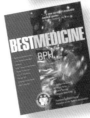
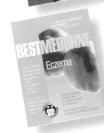
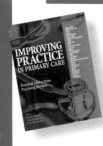
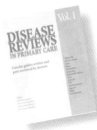
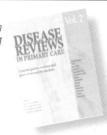
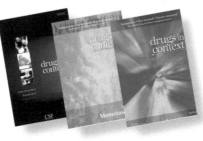